BECOMING REAL:
Harnessing the Power
of Menopause
for Health and Success

With deep regard,

Rose K

BECOMING
REAL

HARNESSING THE POWER
of MENOPAUSE
FOR HEALTH AND SUCCESS

Rose M. Kumar, M.D.

Medial Press • Pewaukee, Wisconsin

Medial Press
www.medial-press.com
www.becoming-real.com
www.ommanicenter.com
The Ommani Center for Integrative Medicine
1166 Quail Court, Suite 210
Pewaukee, WI 53072

ISBN: 978-0-9833521-3-6

Cover design by Dunn+Associates, www.dunn-design.com
Interior design by Dorie McClelland, www.springbookdesign.com

Printed in the United States of America

This book is dedicated to
my daughter, Nisha, and my son, Matthew.
May you always live from Truth and Integrity and
honor only what is Real.
With my love to you forever.

—Mom

Contents

List of figures

Acknowledgments

This book has been a threshold as it emerged in the "middle of my life." The process leading up to its conception and birth has been nothing short of alchemical. I have been burned in many fires which have honed my soul and my truth. My journey has been shared by many who have midwifed my process. Without their guidance, I would not have been able to become "real" to the degree that I have. It is impossible for me to name all of them. I will be forever grateful for their love and support.

My parents, Adarsh and Mahendra Kumar, have been great role models and mentors. Their commitment to integrity, truth, and hard work has had a profound impact on my character and resilience. Their generous gifts throughout my life will carry forward into our future generations as their legacy. Their love and support through my midlife process is one of the reason's I am standing in this real and sacred place.

I thank my beautiful children, Nisha and Matthew, for their unconditional love and their ability to see truth hidden beneath illusion. Because of their resilience, their eagerness to strive for integrity, and their desire to make a positive contribution to our world, I have been empowered to continue to do the same.

My husband, Jerry, is the angel who swept me off my feet in midlife, and continues to support what is real for me. With him, I am learning about the power of living harmoniously with the Feminine and Masculine Principles in relationship, and discovering what *true love* really means. Thank you for your endless support during the writing process and the sacrifices you have so willingly made in order for me to complete this book.

I thank my stepchildren, Hannah and Nicholas, for their love and belief in me and for embracing the path of transformation as we have grown together as a blended family.

I must acknowledge my animal companions, Jazmine, Starlight and Sunbeam, who have silently and powerfully supported me with their unconditional love and loyalty.

My spiritual mentor, Venessa Rahlston, of Soul Genesis, has been invaluable to my transformation. She has helped me reframe my relationship with life by facilitating the integration of my voice, my truth and my power as a woman. She has helped expand my perspective through the window of my soul and has held powerful and unconditional space for my alchemy.

My teacher and guide, Diane Herold, aligned my electrical system through her expertise in energy medicine and taught me the value of boundaries and the intrinsic power of my "real self."

My practice manager at The Ommani Center, Sherris Corby, arrived in my life at a critical time, and helped me reconstruct the Center in the midst of its transmutation. She has been an invaluable friend, and a "big sister." Her dedication to my vision, her expertise as a manager, and her attention to details are an eternal gift to my life's work for which I am deeply grateful. Her love and expertise have been invaluable in the publication of this book.

My friend, Margaret, appeared as a fellow traveler when I began the writing process. Her gift of healing as an energy worker kept me grounded. Her love and enduring friendship have been a constant source of support through my rebirthing.

My business coach, Zeke Lopez, has been an asset to my creative process. He encouraged me to write about my passion and truth in order to share it with the world. His guidance, expertise, and "high intelligence," both intellectually and emotionally, have been gifts throughout my process.

This book itself led me to two gifted people in the publishing industry, Kathi Dunn and Hobie Hobart, of Dunn + Associates

Design, who resonated with my intention and desire to publish a high-quality book. I am grateful for their passion and expertise in helping materialize my written words into the form you are holding in your hands.

My book designer, Dorie McClelland, deserves special and heartfelt acknowledgement for her expertise, patience and ethical principles. She has profoundly influenced my growth as a writer.

I would like to thank Robyn Conley and Maggie Rollins for assisting me in the editing process.

All of the practitioners and staff at The Ommani Center for Integrative Medicine who loyally and faithfully serve the vision of the Center with heart and dedication are deserving of deep gratitude and acknowledgement. Without them, The Ommani Center could not be a reality.

And last but not least, I would like to acknowledge my patients—past, present, and future—who make my life's work possible and who have courageously taught me how to assist in their healing, and use my tools and skills wisely as their physician. I am forever indebted to their offerings of truth and love that bring purpose and meaning to my life's work.

This writing journey awakened my Muse who chose to write this book's contents through me. She was restless and passionate throughout the writing process. I have felt like Her scribe. She took residence in my heart and did not rest until our work was completed. I am amazed at Her intensity.

I am deeply grateful to the Feminine and Masculine energies of the Universe as they continually and precisely manifest themselves on the path leading towards wholeness. I am continually awed by the majesty and constancy of their energies as they patiently and continually teach me what it means to live from heart and soul.

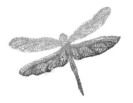

Dragonfly Medicine

Dragonfly is a symbol that represents our ability to discern illusion from reality. We are conditioned to believe we are less powerful than we are. The medicine to heal this wound is Dragonfly Medicine.

It is said Dragonfly was once a mighty dragon with magical powers who was tricked into believing she was a tiny dragonfly. Dragon changed form into a tiny dragonfly due to this false belief.

Too often we believe our failures, our shortcomings and our limitations are real. We are conditioned to believe we are less powerful than we really are. We accept this illusion as our Real self. We need to remember we have a choice to transform and grow into who we really are. We can wield our great inner power and wisdom to change our beliefs about ourselves and transform into our Real selves. When we are able to do this, we heal with the guidance of Dragonfly Medicine.*

My blessing to all who read this book is for you to grow and heal into becoming your Real selves through the Dragonfly Medicine that graces these pages.

May you bless the world as you reconnect with your wisdom and power.

~Rose M. Kumar M.D.

*adapted with permission from Sharon George
www.fantasy-goddess-art.com

1

Uncovering the Feminine

This book was birthed from a deep place of soul. Its birth has been a life's work, born of suffering, reflection and transformation for over half a lifetime. Transformation changes us into larger versions of ourselves. Through transformation, we grow eyes inside of us that enable us to see through the darkness and the fog of illusion into reality.

My heart has always longed for a world that lived from love and compassion, one where health and relationships were inclusive of the feminine qualities of collaboration and process, transformation and balance—one in which truth could be freely expressed and where the voice of integrity was honored as a core value. As a physician, I searched for the presence of these qualities within our health care system. I worked within corporate health care after completing my medical training. I tried all the ways that I could to fit into this system without compromise, but was unable to without paying a grave price. The price was the compromise of my soul's connection to medicine's sacred vocation. True service to its vocation was missing in corporate health care. The corporate environment lacked the Feminine Principle. It lacked all the qualities of the feminine that I cherished, such as, collaborating, loving, listening, healing and feeling. These missing elements were like oxygen for my heart. Without their presence, I was unable to practice the medicine I loved from a place of soul.

I spent my childhood in India, a country where color, stories and myths are important elements of the cultural fabric and where the Goddess is worshipped and revered. As my perspective matured, I realized that I was living in a paradox in this culture which on one hand, spiritualized the feminine, and on the other, suppressed and repressed women. I was unable to understand the reasons for this and could not find an explanation for the dissonance. It seemed hypocritical to me. How could people revere the feminine they projected on to the Goddess and treat women with disrespect? How could they tout the spiritual principles honoring the feminine, yet dismiss the needs of women? My family expected me to conform to these cultural norms, despite my doubts and questions about this paradox. I was suspect if I questioned it.

During my medical training in the U.S., I witnessed the same dissonance. I observed that women in medicine were treated in contrast to the principles of equality. I saw women adapting to this in order to be accepted by the medical system. I saw women patients being dismissed by their doctors if their histories contained emotions or feelings. The feminine qualities of heart and soul were also missing in other organizations across America. I realized that this was a global wound that transcended cultural differences. Its outward appearance differed, but those affected by it suffered similar symptoms of the illness it caused.

The feminine in medicine

As an employee of corporate health care, I witnessed many ways in which the feminine was dishonored. This was both covertly and overtly prevalent, yet it did not seem to be an obvious problem for women in medicine. They were adapting to this treatment and blind to the pain it was causing. Some were angry, but most felt paralyzed. For them, being blind was easier than rocking the boat. When I first joined corporate health care after residency, many women in medicine were becoming intolerant of this injustice and demanding equal treatment. I felt passionate about advocating for the rights of women, and took a stand on our behalf. I advocated for them through the channels that were available in order to improve their condition and made a difference.

My ability to advocate for respect in my personal life was in sharp contrast to my professional life. At home, I had no voice, and was conditioned to second-guess myself and my truth. This part of my life was dissonant with my integrity as a woman who honored the Feminine Principle and practiced it at work. Often, at home, when I requested respect and honor, I was dismissed and undermined. I felt powerless in my attempts to change these dynamics and adapted to them for survival, going blind to the pain that they caused similar to my colleagues at work. I was experiencing the disempowerment that one feels while adapting to the "power principle." I found myself disconnected from my real self at home, yet able to live from it at work. My life was out of balance. I was living in a paradox. Since I was imprinted to not question dissonance, I continued to second-guess myself and felt anguish for how I was dishonored. I thought that somehow I was the cause of the mistreatment I was receiving.

I needed to heal the disparity between my personal and professional lives. Since there was dissonance between them, I felt tossed between two worlds—one in which I had clarity around how women deserved to be treated, and one where I felt intense fear and resistance. I began a process to evaluate and understand why I felt anguish in my personal life. I had to become conscious of the behaviors and treatment that I was adapting to and the reasons why I was. This was the beginning of my recovery process.

Personal recovery opened my eyes to what was really happening to many women in medicine. I noticed that they reluctantly adapted to a system that left them with little to no connection with what was real in order to survive. Although I had strongly advocated on their behalf, my personal process opened a deeper perspective within me regarding their dishonor in the medical system. They also treated *themselves* with dishonor by compromising their truth in order to be accepted, which was clearly a factor in how the system treated them. I had done the same in my personal life. These adapted patterns became clear to me as my inner-eyes opened. I was finally able to see through the fog of illusion into the reality of my situation.

I observed that the medical system often caused women, both patients and physicians, to second-guess themselves as they adapted to patterns of treatment that dishonored both them and their process. This system was neither heart centered nor respectful to the true ethics and integrity of medicine. It did not serve the soul or the vocation of health care. On the contrary, it perpetuated a fear-based system that disempowered all.

Integrative medicine

Integrative medicine was becoming a new buzz word. It seemed like a better approach to health which was confirmed by health care data. It made sense to integrate complementary (alternative) and traditional medicine. It appeared to be a more complete model for health care. The medical system began to open clinics that offered both traditional and complementary medicine and called it integrative medicine. The intent of this form of medicine was logical in theory, and corporate health care wanted to capture market share. Patients began swarming to these clinics with the expectation of humanistic less fragmented and less pathologically focused health care. Over a relatively short period of time, most left disappointed, as they experienced the traditional model practiced beneath a new label, one that still saw illness as a break in the body that could be fixed through "alternative" rather than traditional means. Focus on the *causes* of illness was still not a part of this system. Experiencing a potpourri of modalities in conjunction with traditional symptom management provided only a limited level of healing, as it was unable to provide an understanding of cause and therefore *true* healing. Patients continued to feel disempowered within this new model. They found that this form of medicine was not truly integrative, but was a traditional medical model that used complementary medicine from its limited framework. They were actually spending even more money for alternative methods in addition to traditional ones for symptomatic relief.

In addition, around this time, a number of "holistic" doctors emerged in an effort to meet these needs, but many they were not utilizing standard of care and were implementing medical practices that were not safe, nor scientifically proven to be effective. Sometimes they did more harm than good. Patients were still searching for a better and more effective way to heal and the open system they sought was not found in either traditional or integrative medicine within the current health care model.

I was becoming increasingly restless as I felt the critical and meaningful essence of healing missing in health care. I felt that the current medical model was too limited to truly heal. I began to envision a health care model that would be invested in healing rather than merely symptom management; where the Feminine Principle, when integrated, could heal the health care system itself. This would also have the potential to heal the deep wound of feminine suffering apparent in corporate health care.

It was time to create a health care model that honored the vocation of medicine, one that was inclusive of process and committed to educating patients. I felt that the medical system needed to reintegrate the Feminine Principle at all levels of its infrastructure, both as a business and a medical model. This was the crucial missing piece in the corporate health care. I began to realize that my life's work was to create a medical model that included the qualities of collaboration, listening, feeling and expertise. It would not compromise standard of care in favor of the Feminine Principle. It would be inclusive of both. This could reframe health care into a working model where its intent and mission included the facilitation of wholeness. This would be truly integrative.

I attempted to practice medicine from this perspective within corporate health care. The response from management was not encouraging. They felt threatened by this "open system" of practice. They asked me to down play my approach and accommodate what was familiar and normal for the current system—sick care. They informed me that they would not support a medical practice that did not maintain sickness, as it compromised hospital dollars. Supporting health did not work for their business model which relied on costly diagnostic procedures and hospital admissions. My low admission numbers were not matching their projected profits as my patients were maintaining health. Patients were healing in my practice. This was a conflict of interest for the system. I was disheartened. But, I was not willing to compromise my soul to increase their quarterly profits.

I left corporate health care to create a new medical model, one where I could practice what I loved: a form of medicine that maintained traditional standard of care and *healed* its patients. It would integrate the wisdom and expertise of traditional medicine with the wisdom of complementary healing traditions that had been scientifically proven. I felt that this could reframe the current health care model and transform it into one that could heal patients with both the scientific expertise of traditional medicine and well established disciplines of complementary medicine. It would not substitute scientifically based traditional methods with complementary methods. This framework would also be inclusive of the Feminine Principle. This would offer patients the experience of a medical system that offered validation and empowerment as they made their journeys through life's difficulties. Patients would be able to make sense of their suffering within this inclusive framework. As they learned to live from heart and meaning, they would be able to reclaim themselves. I felt that I needed to create this medical model in order to practice medicine that was both scientific and heart centered. This was my deepest calling.

The process of creating this model was itself a powerful "medicine" in my recovery from working in corporate health care. At its foundation, it contained the elements of both the Masculine and Feminine Principles. Both were needed for *true* healing. High standard of care would be maintained in the search for the *causes* of illness. These causes created the symptoms that my traditional medical tools could fix. I found that when patients uncovered these causes, their health improved as they integrated their awareness into making healthier life choices. This prevented the recurrence of their symptoms and future illnesses. It also made them self-responsible. This form of health care would offer education and the exploration of process, where both biology and biography were considered as critical components in healing and standard of care was not compromised. This model could evoke the seeker in patients—where their curiosity could guide them to the answers they sought. This could deepen their experience of life. Illness could be their catalyst to awaken. This health care model could also facilitate awakening and transforming *before* a life crisis occurred by teaching patients how to live more consciously. This could prevent illness. This could connect patients to their intrinsic power and wisdom. This model could awaken consciousness.

This could be a way to serve people that were asking for a more patient-centered model of health care, and could reform the current ailing medical system at foundational levels. A health care system based on the integration of the process oriented Feminine Principle of healing, balanced with the expertise oriented Masculine Principle of fixing, was a model that I believed, could restore the soul of medicine, the soul that had been buried underneath the mechanical and heartless system that medicine had become.

This health care model also needed to be a healthy business that was not willing to compromise care for profit. Unlike the business of health care today, this business would be sustainable, ecological, profitable and cost effective while operating from the soul of the vocation of medicine.

I realized this was my opportunity to recalibrate my life's work.

My personal recovery had uncovered a powerful turn in my life. In this manner, the reclamation and healing from abuse in my personal life could serve as a catalyst for healing health care, where the feminine was also undermined and neglected, disrespected and dismissed. The soul of medicine was still alive, but buried underneath the corporate, closed and disempowering framework. It was time to bring heart centered care to the medical system and create a medical model that restored the sacred back into its vocation.

Open and closed systems

Therapist and author, Virginia Satir, categorizes systems as being either closed or open. A system consists of individual parts that are essential and related to one another. These parts interact to serve a goal or a purpose according to rules determined by the system. Power distributed amongst a few members is necessary to maintain the working of the system's components in order to deal with influences from the outside.

In a *closed system,* the ones in power separate it from outside interference and influence in order to maintain its internal dynamic. This maintains the system's "status quo." The operating principle in this system determines that *performance* defines the worth of its members. The "power principle" is constantly working to make sure that the rules of the system are being followed and its members receive negative consequences for not following them. These rules are made by a few members in power within the closed system.

An *open system* is one in which intrinsic worth is of prime value. Performance is related to it, but it does not define it. Change within the system is welcomed and is a normal part of its growth. In fact, it is desirable. Communication is an important element in an open system that keeps its dynamics healthy.

Lack of communication is the hallmark of a closed system. In closed systems, people are uncommunicative and defensive when they are questioned. Secrecy is the unwritten rule, and a lack of trust is prevalent among its members.

Often, when people are second-guessing themselves and feel fearful, confused or disempowered, they are interacting within a closed system. A closed system does not communicate in order to clarify intent or interact from integrity or truth. Its focus is to maintain its rules, the "status quo."

Many of us can agree that we grew up in closed systems. The "code of conduct" was determined by the people in power and we adapted to the rules of the system. The larger system that influenced the family was the cultural system within which the family existed. Questioning unhealthy cultural norms was often not permitted within the family. The family can become a closed system if it follows the rules and code of conduct normalized by the culture's closed system. Open communication is not present and problem solving is not valued. Rules are followed to maintain the system's status quo.

I lived within in a closed system as a child and then in my personal relationship as an adult. When I questioned the unhealthy dynamics that I was expected to normalize, I was silenced. At that time, I had no understanding of the concepts described here. The most prevalent feeling I lived with was fear. It kept me from feeling safe and having trust within relationships. In my relationship as an adult, I frequently walked on eggshells, afraid of the punitive consequences I would suffer when I communicated my needs and longings for the system to grow and evolve. I was living within a closed system in my personal life, where I had no power, no voice, and was adapting to it with learned behaviors from the closed system I was raised in.

By my forties, I was unwilling to continue to live from what felt familiar, but was unhealthy. I needed to reconfigure my relationship to myself. I needed to reclaim my personal and intrinsic authority to re-evaluate myself through my heart and feelings. I knew when I was not being true to myself and what I needed in order to experience integrity and self-respect. As a child I had been taught that I had no intrinsic authority to assert my will, and that my instincts were wrong. This was reinforced in my personal relationship as an adult and also by the medical system where I received my training. I was taught, as many of us are, to override my instincts and my inner voice in order to conform to the rules defined by the closed system that I lived in. I did not feel any differences between the closed systems of my culture, my personal life or health care. All evoked fear and punitive consequences when the rules were questioned. There was no room for growth or change. I adapted to this framework in order to survive. It made me vulnerable to abuse. I second-guessed myself frequently as the result of my cultural and familial imprinting. My relationships to my intuition, my instinct and my inner wisdom were all wounded. I did not feel safe in my own skin.

Are physicians and patients the victims of a closed system of health care?

In the twenty-five years that I have been a part of the medical system, I have observed a consistent truth about physicians. A majority of them chose their careers in medicine in order to help and heal others. They entered the medical system in order to serve the vocation of medicine. The framework from which the corporate medical system operates sets physicians up for adapting to the closed system of health care. They leave their medical training in significant debt, as well as, severely fatigued from long hours at work and lack of sleep for nearly a decade. They are wounded by the adaptations needed for surviving their long and difficult training. They complete their residencies and seek employment as a means to pay off their debts, regain balance and utilize their learned skill sets as physicians. If they are employed by corporate health care, they quickly realize that it requires them to conform to the next and new set of rules of its closed system. Questioning these would lead to punitive consequences. Since they are conditioned to adapt, they compromise their souls for security.

When we adapt to closed systems that are based in fear, we often incorporate its elements into our behaviors. Since fear disempowers us, we unconsciously project it onto others, attempting to compensate for our loss of personal power. When we do this, fear becomes a part of our energy field and permeates our lives in both subtle and overt ways. When we are fearful, we often evoke fear in others. The majority of physicians who work within the current system of health care are fearful. The conditions of medical practice today evoke fear, and the rules of the closed system of corporate health care also evoke fear. Patients are almost always fearful when they go to see their physicians. Fear is the primary feeling within the current health care system. It clearly signals that both physicians and patients are members of a closed system.

Is the current health care system a closed system?

The Feminine Principle approaches relationships from dynamics of connection and collaboration. It is able to bear witness for others and hold space for truth and feelings. Behaving from these qualities requires courage and fierceness. Speaking one's truth without the fear of rejection is an act of fierceness.

In a closed system, codependency is the operating principle in relationships between its members. A few members, in positions of power and authority, have domination over subordinate members who adapt to being dominated, and compromise their truth and sovereignty to maintain the system's internal dynamic. Dominators require subordinates to dominate, and subordinates are conditioned to adapt to being dominated. This dynamic wounds and disempowers people. The elements of the "power principle" that dominators employ regulates behavior through fear and control. In this dynamic, intrinsic power is not accessible, and collaboration is not valued. The system's goal is to maintain its status quo. If members within this system begin to outgrow its dysfunctional dynamics and relate from a place of health, other members of the system often react and attempt to manipulate the subordinate into behaving from familiar unhealthy dynamics. Their intent is to maintain the system's status quo. Members are unable to trust those in authority, and walk on eggshells compromising their truth and their needs. They do this in order to avoid conflict if they are too afraid to leave the system. Over time, this pattern becomes the governing dynamic between its members. It becomes incorporated into their psyches and behaviors. They become blind to healthy behaviors. All of their relationships operate from the dynamics of a closed system. This dynamic is prevalent in corporate health care.

In an *open* system, its members can be true to themselves and feel assured that they will be treated with respect and honor as long as they behave from integrity. Self-responsibility is a core element present within relationships in an open system. The system stays open to growth and change and its participants grow within it and with it as it evolves. As members seek their own health, the system grows healthy. This is the kind of system I longed for. I had not experienced relationships like this in my training, as an employee of corporate health care or my personal life. I did not have a relative position from which to choose healthy relationships. However, I intrinsically knew and felt that relationships could exist from this open dynamic. This felt healthy. The presence of this dynamic within any system could evoke health. I believed this open system was needed in corporate health care.

The Ommani Center for Integrative Medicine

After many years of working within corporate health care, I realized that for this system, true *health* was a conflict of interest; it didn't generate hospital profits. As people stayed healthy, hospital admissions, diagnostic and pharmaceutical interventions all decreased. This did not serve the health care system's financial objectives. It threatened them. An open system of healing could not function within the closed system of corporate health care if it relied on the sickness of patients. I realized I had to leave this system in order to practice true health care. I needed to create an open system of health care that resonated with the soul of my vocation.

I created The Ommani Center for Integrative Medicine as a prototype of an open system of health care. Its vision was committed to health, education and transformation. Medicine practiced from this framework quickly began to heal its community of patients. This open system was in stark contrast to the closed system of corporate health care that I had left.

A few years after establishing The Ommani Center, I awakened to the reality in which I was living. I was living in a closed system in my personal life. I had adapted to this and had gone blind and numb to how disempowered I felt. I was living the familiar paradox of my childhood and my cultural conditioning. At this juncture, I could not function in an open system at work and live in a closed system at home. The Ommani Center was created on the principles of transformation and wholeness and required me to live its vision authentically. Soon after I awakened to this, my personal life imploded, marking my midlife gateway.

After years of being treated with disrespect and dishonor, my personal relationship hit a new low. This activated my midlife transformational process. I had to face the blindness that resulted from my adapted state. I needed to examine all the ways that I had tried to maintain "stability" by remaining compliant. I needed to dismantle my negative self-talk and conditioned way of being that caused me to adapt to dishonor and disrespect. This was my opportunity to reweave myself and reconstruct a life of health and honor that resonated with the Feminine Principle. I had a responsibility to dismantle the degradation of the feminine, and powerfully redefine and reintegrate her into my life. This was my midlife juncture point. This was my task at hand.

After I filed for divorce, I found myself in the midst of the energy and chaos of an intense death-and-rebirth cycle. I needed to create a new life from the rubble of the old. I needed to find a path to transform and to transmute myself from an adapted woman who tolerated abuse, into a woman who lived from self-respect and "walked her talk." I needed to embody this as my work was committed to the facilitation of true healing. Through this gateway, I needed to reclaim my integrity and self-worth and reframe my relationship to my intrinsic self and align it with the vision of the open system of health care that I had created.

Through this process, I realized the immense responsibility that we all have in midlife. This gateway expects much of us. The journey I undertook would not only be valuable for me, but for my children, my patients and everyone I would encounter. It would connect me more deeply with my life's work. Only by courageously aligning myself with this process could I earn the trust of the women and men who relied on me for guidance. They were seeking a path through the treacherous territories of their own gateways. They were seeking a way to transform their compensated and adapted selves into their real selves. Unless I knew this territory and navigated my way through it to become real, I myself would not have the insight to guide them; in fact it could be dangerous for them to entrust me to help them through their process if I was unaware of the terrain.

When I realized that my inner work required this level of personal transformation, I discovered the voluminous amounts of material that had been written about this process. In fact, I had been collecting books and articles on this topic of midlife for five years prior to this juncture point. My instinct had already been helping me without my conscious awareness, and preparing me for what was to come. This material was my solace and offered me much needed guidance. In addition, mentors appeared in my life that midwifed and oriented me through my journey. I had an insatiable hunger to rediscover myself and to dismantle all of my parts that were compensated, adapted and inauthentic. My intent for recovery and reclamation manifested a safe container within which I could heal and be supported as I engaged in this difficult, powerful and deeply intense work. It provided me with solace and safety through the terror of deconstruction that my identity was experiencing and that my soul expected me to undergo.

Looking back over the years, I could see that a theme had been prevalent throughout my personal and professional lives. I had frequently felt profound loneliness which I was not able to understand or satisfy. As I underwent my transformative process, I began to see it as the pain of separation from the Feminine Principle. Loneliness was a symptom of my disconnection from the feminine as I adapted to the closed systems of which I had been a part. I needed to reintegrate the Feminine Principle into my life. I began to see all the ways in which our collective culture was dismissive of the sacred feminine and how we all participated. If our world was beckoning a paradigm shift, then healing this wound was necessary. As I reconstructed my identity to include elements of Feminine Principle, I was able to reframe all of my relationships to include respect, honor, love and integrity. This healed my relationship to the sacred feminine. It also enabled me to practice medicine authentically.

When we awaken to our inner truth through suffering caused by deep wounds, we regain the inner sight we previously denied ourselves, resulting from our fear of being rejected by others. We need our inner sight to access our intrinsic power. The price we pay for our blindness is enormous and grave. The midlife process does not support this blind way of being. The relationships that we choose to stay blind to invariably fail us. We suffer deep wounding through this alchemical process of "failure." The blessing from the deep wound is the powerful "medicine" it holds. This medicine permeates our lives and graces us with the clarity of vision that can no longer be fooled by adaptations or cover-ups. This

medicine reconnects us to our real selves and reveals the vulner-
abilities that we carry that have conditioned us to adapt and compromise our truth. Once we awaken to this, we are able to reclaim
our intrinsic power.

The value of being heart centered

Our heart is the seat of truth, honor, integrity and love, yet in
today's world, we do not live from it. These healthy elements have
been replaced by competition and entitlement resulting in duality
and separation from one another. A framework based on duality
contains dynamics that evoke separation. It operates from concepts
based on "either or" or "us versus them" beliefs. When these concepts define our dynamics, they result in violent and painful behaviors with outcomes visible on the daily news. Interacting from them
weakens us at deep levels as they lack the heart-centered qualities of
the Feminine Principle. This has been prevalent for many centuries
and has caused great suffering.

The heart does not relate through duality. On the contrary,
it relates through interpersonal connection and collaboration.
Unification is always its intent. The heart is unable to operate from
"either or," and "us versus them" concepts that our culture normalizes. The heart operates from inclusive "both and" concepts. This
is the heart's natural state. The heart resonates with open systems.
The heart aches when duality is the operating principle. Duality
generates fear; unity generates love. Love is powerful, resilient,
fierce and uncompromising. However, our culture defines love
differently. Its definition confuses codependency for love. This
cultural definition is based on the dynamics of closed systems. We
have normalized these distortions. We must redefine and reframe
our definition of love to include the strong elements of the Feminine Principle. We need to restore our cultural definition to its
original and purest root.

As we awaken to the power present in fierce love, and begin to behave from it, our lives feel miraculous. When we live from distortions and replace what is real with a façade, we pay a heavy price. We only do this when we adapt from conditioned behaviors. The powerful elements of the Feminine Principle that are necessary for our health and happiness lay buried underneath this façade. By midlife, living from adaptation begins to feel empty and superficial. It no longer brings us happiness. When we awaken to this, we feel disillusioned. Disillusionment is painful but through it, we are can begin to see and feel more clearly. We can see the reality buried underneath the heavy illusions in our world. Our society, as a whole, lives in accordance to the rules of a closed system. This results in our disconnection from the sacred feminine which leads to loneliness and loss of meaning in our lives. It takes courage and endurance to reintegrate the feminine into our relationships with our selves. This is our holy task through midlife.

The medial place

It takes great courage and endurance to swim upstream, to not feel like a victim and to connect to and live from one's real self. Story teller and Jungian analyst, Dr. Clarissa Pinkole Estes, describes midlife as the "medial place." It is the midpoint in our lives when we release the "world of expectations" in favor of the "world of soul." It is the gateway between the ages of 42 and 49 where we have to choose between what feels familiar but adapted (for which we compromise our truth), and what feels real and resonates with our truth. This medial place necessitates honesty and courage in order for us to make important and powerful choices. We must choose to live from our truth and enter the world of soul. This is a paradigm shift in midlife, an initiation necessary for our journey to wholeness. This gateway holds the potential to transform our lives into ones with more heart and meaning. Our world itself is in a gateway, a "medial place." Our normalized and adapted ways of being are no longer working. We must choose to collectively live from soul as we pass through this gateway.

Midlife crisis and Women's Health redefined

If the closed system of corporate health care defines Women's Health today, we cannot expect it to heal us, or even offer us direction through midlife.

As women enter midlife, they straddle the time between perimenopause (the time surrounding menopause) and menopause. The health care system sees this transition through its lens of pathology and physicians diligently attempt to cover the symptoms that accompany it. Menopause is viewed as an illness, a disease of hormone deficiency, not the powerful transformational process that it is. The traditional health care system negates process and finds ways to numb out and dumb down feeling function and the emotive qualities of women. It dismisses the questions they ask about themselves and their changing bodies as their powerful midlife process unfolds and they seek ways to reclaim themselves and their sense of worth from the culture that continues to disempower them.

Corporate health care is unable to meet their needs. The numbers of hysterectomies, synthetic hormone prescriptions, antidepressants and sleep-aids climax in midlife women. The health care system has defined its protocol as 'treat and medicate' in order to eliminate symptoms of perimenopause and menopause. Symptom control is big business for health care. Physicians are not allowed to question these treatments and many physicians are required to fulfill quotas of diagnostic tests and surgical procedures in order to maintain their employment within the corporate health care system. The field of Women's Health suffers a deep soul loss at the hands of these protocols within this closed system, and the midlife process loses its power and purpose when women are pharmaceutically numbed and their process is dismissed. As a result, women begin to second-guess themselves and fear their process.

Midlife and the health care system

Midlife is a time when we must listen to our longings and inner callings and follow them with soulfulness and integrity. This has the power to restore self-worth and self-respect. Currently, our society does not have a framework in order to facilitate this. This would require an open system within which we can live and grow. If our organizations were open systems, they would be supportive of the transformational process evoked by our changing bodies. They would help us to evolve and grow during this gateway that offers us a second chance to live from our authenticity and truth. They would be committed to our health through the "medial place." We would be guided and supported as we dismantled our adapted and fearful selves and transformed our lives into ones that evoked depth and meaning.

This gateway is a time when we must begin asking the deeper and crucial questions about our worth and our purpose in life. In order for the health care system to facilitate this process, it must transform into open system to support health and transformation. Biological manipulation and symptom management alone do not fulfill a woman's needs through this gateway. Closed systems, like corporate health care, currently do not offer support for personal growth. Instead, they mask and control the physical symptoms that can catalyze personal growth. We must understand the biological causes of physical symptoms in addition to the deeper questions they evoke in order to facilitate intrinsic health and uncover meaning in midlife.

Why is the menopausal transition so difficult for women in America? Why do we experience menopausal symptoms in epidemic proportions? How can women safely transform through their midlife transitions? How can they be intrinsically empowered and not dismissed with synthetic hormones and psychiatric medications?

As a physician, I am awed by the physiology of menopause. It is biologically precise and has common elements that all women share. In this book, I have explored these physical aspects in addition to uncovering the inner life of the midlife woman. She begins to feel her truth and power arise within her through feelings that facilitate her connection to her real self. This is illustrated through stories of midlife women and how their symptoms and processes created a "course correction" where they were able to step away from an adapted to a more authentic path with guidance from their intense feelings, instincts and intuitions. I have also presented my framework of the "Four Body System." This framework provides an understanding of how symptoms that present at physical and mental levels may have their origins at emotional and energetic levels. An understanding of these levels is important so that one can seek the appropriate care needed for healing. This can accelerate the restoration of well-being on the journey towards true health and wholeness in midlife.

Women's Health is currently defined by our traditional medical system through a lens of pathology. I have replaced this with a transformational lens, where it becomes evident that an open system for healthy transformation and balance is critical for safe guidance through the territory of midlife. I have presented many stories of courage and healing from women's lives—ordinary, midlife women like you and me. During their midlife transitions, these women redefined and reframed themselves from feeling like victims to feeling empowered and free.

As midlife women, we have an immense and important opportunity to help our hurting world. Our world-systems need to transform from closed into open ones in order to heal the chaos and separation that has created suffering for all. Facilitating this transformation will require our collective effort.

My hope is that this book will awaken us to question our normalized, unhealthy and adapted lives that long for meaning, and encourage us to redefine our understanding of health. We need to heal the cultural wounds that perpetuate the *illusion* of health and integrate and live from its true definition. We need to engage our courage to transform our closed systems into open ones committed to growth and empowerment. This powerful work transcends race, color, religion, gender and nationality. It is the sacred and true work of our time.

My intent is to evoke creative thought which facilitates us to question the "status quo" as defined by the current and prevailing paradigm of the "power principle" whose presence is central to maintaining our current closed systems. Our questioning is necessary for both our personal and organizational health and healing.

My hope is to encourage the beginning of a dialogue that can transform our current definition of Women's Health which does not value empowerment or feeling function, into one that is inclusive of these elements. At its heart, this redefinition will be restorative and healing, and acknowledge the death-and-life cycle of transformation as a necessary part of our personal and collective growth. This redefinition can only occur by reintegrating the Feminine Principle into our relationships and our current systems.

This courageous and necessary work has the potential to heal the deep wounds in our culture and transform the shape and feeling of our personal and professional lives. Ultimately, this could also transform our health care system into one we can trust again for our healing.

2

What Is Real?

Becoming Real

At 45, I awaken a weaver-
I weave soul into substance.
As my old self falls away,
I take up strong thread and
weave myself anew.
For me, it was marked;
I was hollowed out.
I needed this to resurrect,
to live,
to thrive.
For some, it is gentle,
for me, it was alchemical.
By turning lead into gold,
it turned a woman of the world
into a woman of Soul.
I felt the deepest pain,
cried tears that didn't stop;
released joy in laughter,
discovered melody in my song.
The tapestry of my heart,
now sewn with stronger thread,
seeps Soul into my Presence.
I am the Medial One,
I have become Real.
I will take the next step.

There is a belief in indigenous mythology that we carry our "double" within our souls. Our "double" is the part of us that forms our "real self," and calls to us to embody it. She does not become tainted by our wounding and provides us with the resilience and strength needed for our healing. She embodies our wholeness. She carries the "codes" for our higher destinies. When we are wounded and sometimes disconnect from our real selves, we may miss Her call and may fail to manifest our higher destinies. The call from our "double" is the loudest during midlife. This is the time when the veil between our unconscious and conscious selves is most porous. When our hormones part and the transition to the second half of life beckons, our souls move closer to us than any other time in our lives. Some of us have not been able to access our truth before this gateway, as we mistakenly identified our wounded selves for our real selves. We are called from within as a reminder that there is more to life than how we have been living. Our "double" carries within Her our deeper and more meaningful life.

Our "double" is always trying to carry us towards our highest destiny. Life often presents us with choices to upgrade or downgrade our course. Midlife is an important gateway where we need to choose between authenticity and familiarity. It takes courage to choose authenticity. When we listen to the call of our "double" and make the choice to connect with our authenticity, we can embody our real selves during the second half of our lives and live from our higher destinies.

Alice

One of my friends, Alice, was a 66-year-old attorney. For many years, she was bedridden with a neurological illness. She told me that while in her forties, she felt that she was in a gateway that presented two doors before her. One was familiar and had the trappings of corporate law that would require her to be ruthless to achieve material success, while the other door felt unfamiliar and led to the unknown. She chose the familiar door with material trappings and walked through it into a career of corporate law. She was successful from society's standards but her life of ruthlessness lacked meaning. She had great regrets for choosing the familiar door. She always wondered what path she had missed behind the other door.

She admitted that she chose the familiar due to her fear of the unknown. During her career, she often wondered what her life would have been like had she chosen the other door. I also wondered what her life would have been like. Would she have been fulfilled and happy? She played the part expected of her and pursued society's definition of success compromising what was real for her. Her soul always longed for more meaning. She spent the last days of her life in regret for having chosen familiarity through her midlife gateway. I will never forget her call to me before she died. She encouraged me to follow my bliss. She asked me to promise her that I would not make the same mistake that she did. She had spent the last 30 years of her life in pursuit of what was not real. She felt this in the depths of her being. Her "double" had been calling to her. She was buried underneath her worldly trappings. In the end, she knew that she had not lived from her highest destiny.

The dismantled feminine

As women, we often make errors in judgment like Alice did, due to our conditioning by society's rules and expectations. We have been doing this for thousands of years. The feminine was dismantled from our world approximately 4000 years ago. Since then, our culture has been wounded. The feminine is at the heart of our instincts and feeling function. We sacrifice feminine qualities of feelings and process in favor of performance and product, as our society devalues feminine qualities. The results of this are evident in our world today. When we turn on our televisions, we bear witness to ourselves in a violent and angry world, bereft of real meaning.

The lack of meaning generates hopelessness and anger within us that we unknowingly project onto others. But anger, as an emotion, can also be used as a catalyst for transformation. It can be used creatively to direct us back onto a more authentic and real path. Anger can be a powerful call to action. It can be used to reclaim wholeness and balance. It can help reconnect us with our truth. Anger can only be effective as a catalyst if we use it consciously with intent to transform. Reactive anger is destructive. When used with consciousness, it can be creative. Our lives are too often driven by the wounds present in our subconscious and unconscious minds. Our unawareness of these wounds can cause us to use anger in destructive ways. Living without awareness can disconnect us from our real selves. The real self is intrinsically powerful. It is the self that is capable of alchemy. It is not contaminated by cultural distortions. If we do not connect with our real selves, we often risk attempting to find meaning by external means. This leaves us with feelings of emptiness and disconnects us from our intrinsic power. In order to compensate for this disconnection we may try to dominate others in false attempts to restore our sense of power and worth. This perpetuates the dysfunctional dynamics that are currently present in our society.

Society has rules and protocols that it expects us to obey in order for it to accept us. While some rules are needed for our safety, many are over-controlling and do not resonate with our real selves because they limit our access to the truth. Additionally, society distorts what it defines as "masculine" or "feminine." Many of society's definitions lack truth and authenticity. For example, society defines success as the accumulation of material wealth. In order to live in accordance with this definition we may need to work long hours, under great stress and sacrifice our relationships. By normalizing this pattern, we may adapt as others do and compromise what is meaningful to us, becoming blind to this dysfunction. We often behave in these ways in order to feel accepted, resulting in the abdication of our true values. If we reject our inner truths for acceptance, we often lose the intrinsic connection with our "double." We may find ourselves justifying our compromises and normalizing them. Many use justifications in order to avoid feelings of loneliness that accompany the disconnection from their real selves.

As we approach midlife, what is normalized by society begins to feel like a façade. Our "double" cannot be fooled. She expresses our disconnection from Her in our feelings of emptiness and lack of meaning that begin to surface in midlife. During this gateway, we have the opportunity to transform and connect with our real selves by listening to Her call which sometimes manifests through our physical and mental symptoms, and we must choose to reconnect to our truth in order to feel whole. This can awaken our creativity and can activate the courage needed to follow our bliss. This can lead us onto our higher destinies.

The midlife journey

The journey in midlife is one that we can all choose to make. Many take this journey unconsciously due our society's lack of framework needed for transformation. For many, midlife is marked with what is called a "midlife crisis." Sometimes, a crisis occurs in order to facilitate our connection with our "double." If we live unconsciously through the first half of our lives, fate often forces us to awaken through a crisis in order to catalyze our need for connection with our real selves. This often becomes the gateway through which we can intrinsically reconstruct our lives. For some the crisis takes the form of an illness, for others, it takes the form of a divorce or the loss of a job or a loved one. For all, it is the call from the "double" to become who we really are beneath our imprinted and adapted selves. In order to dismantle our unhealthy imprints, we need to individuate from familiarity. It is frightening to leave the known behind, but we must in order to redefine ourselves more authentically.

The power of familiarity

We spent the first few decades of our lives in our family systems, and their dynamics imprinted us. We carried these imprints into our relationships as adults. If they were unhealthy or dysfunctional, we risked creating the same or similar dynamics in our adult relationships. Most of us are unconscious of the imprinted patterns we carry. We often attract relationships that remind us of dynamics from our families of origin. These dynamics feel like "home." They feel familiar. We also live from adaptations that we learned in our family systems. Many of us adapted to dysfunctional dynamics in order to feel accepted and to "fit in." Some of these adaptations required us to disconnect from our real selves. When we were young, we did not realize that we were compromising ourselves while doing this. We were conditioned to behave in ways expected of us. Some of these behaviors were necessary for our socialization, but many were not healthy and were adaptations for survival. Since our family was our safety, we adapted in order to survive. As we learned these survival strategies, we moved further away from our real feelings. This often resulted in feelings of loneliness and loss during the first half of our lives. These feelings were difficult to understand. We felt wounded. We often felt invalidated and sometimes not even seen or heard. These feelings often manifested as depression and anxiety.

As midlife approaches, these wounds call for healing. It becomes difficult for many to be around their families of origin during their midlife gateways. I realized this when I noticed many of my midlife patients coming to see me for support before family gatherings. They would come to reinforce their newly discovered truths that had been hidden underneath their adapted selves. They were afraid of losing contact with their connection to their real selves while around their families of origin. Within a few days with their families, they found themselves behaving from the familiar and adapted patterns they learned as children. This caused them to feel stress and anxiety. A sense of relief accompanied the end of the family gathering when they could return to their real selves which resonated with their truth.

The dynamics of familiarity that we recreate during the first half of our lives often resonate with the dynamics of closed systems. In midlife, our souls call us to deconstruct these dynamics, which are adapted and fear-based. This necessitates the creation of open systems within which we our truth can be lived. This offers us a deeper sense of meaning. It takes great courage to live from our truth. We often risk being rejected by others when we undergo the alchemical process through our midlife gateways. As we dismantle adapted and inauthentic behaviors and uncover our real selves, we no longer resonate with others who behave from patterns that we are dismantling. They often reject us. Transforming into our real selves releases our need for external validation and restores our integrity. It also restores our self-reliance and heals our anxiety and low self-worth. It reconnects us with our intrinsic power.

Individuation

Carl Jung was a well-known psychiatrist who coined the term "individuation." Individuation is the process during adolescence and midlife of separating from family of origin and identifying with the real self hidden underneath the familiar and adapted self. This process requires great courage. We are always led through this by our "double." In this process, She awakens our ability to see our unconscious and hidden agendas that are present in our shadows that are based in fear and created from our imprinting with reinforcement from society. This process is frightening, yet powerful. It holds within it the potential to open our inner-eyes. It exposes the rules and operating principles we may be unconsciously living from. It requires us to dismantle those that are inauthentic. It is profoundly difficult to do this in adolescence, especially since our society lacks framework to facilitate this process. Many adults in our society are not individuated and are unable to guide adolescents safely through their individuations. In Indigenous cultures, individuated mentors take adolescents on vision quests where they are led through a series of rituals in order to make contact with their "double" and gain wisdom and insight from Her. These adolescents are then able to incorporate the wisdom gained into their lives and unfold their higher destinies with consciousness awakened through this process. This process is viewed as an initiation and is considered deeply sacred. It can only be facilitated by mentors who have transformed into their real selves and know the territory of this initiation.

Our society sadly lacks awareness around the power and purpose of this process. In our culture, we often pass through the gateways of adolescence and midlife unconsciously and attempt to fill our emptiness with superficial and material trappings. Many of us currently in midlife had the chance to individuate in adolescence, but due to the lack of mentorship, we may have missed out on connecting with our real selves during that gateway. In midlife, we get a second chance to individuate and connect with our real selves.

The complacency in our society towards living unconsciously endangers our individuation. We normalize our adapted ways of living and often medicate our emptiness. The price we pay for this is soul loss. In these ways, we often lose contact with our truth and sovereignty. We need to reevaluate our choices and use the midlife gateway as our opportunity to transform and individuate. This is the sacred task of our generation. This can lead to the restoration of a deeper sense of meaning and self-respect. In fact, it can have a profound effect on future generations. It may even heal many of the challenges we face today that result from our attempts to solve society's problems with ineffective and superficial solutions. These are often a result of our lack of individuation.

Our motivation to unfold our real selves and support each other to do the same has the potential to restore the health of our culture in profound ways. The field of Women's Health must be redefined to include support and guidance through individuation as a necessary part of its framework. In order for women to bring transformational solutions to our world, they need to connect with their intrinsic power and wisdom. Women's Health has a responsibility to facilitate the reconnection of women with their real selves through their midlife gateways. When offered from this framework, Women's Health can have a significant impact on the healing of society at large.

The dilemma in parenting

We have experienced how our imprinting has impacted our destiny tracks and our sense of meaning and fulfillment. When we remain unindividuated, we are not able to relate to our children from adult behaviors that are necessary to facilitate their movement towards their higher destinies. When we are unindividuated as parents we may unconsciously expect our children's choices to fulfill *our* unmet needs. We can get caught in the loop of using *their* performance to define *our* self-worth. We are often unaware that this is our projection. It is heavily influenced by our culture and our conditioning, as well as, our adapted selves that we may have mistaken for our real selves. When we do this, our children feel the imposition of our projections and often rebel against our expectations if they do not resonate with them. If they are punished into fulfilling them, they risk losing contact with their truth and their real selves. They risk losing access to the voice of their "double." They risk integrating our projections into their thought patterns and being intrinsically controlled by them. In this way, we risk perpetuating our adapted patterns onto our children. Awareness of this is necessary for parents of adolescents. For those of us in midlife, we must realize how we were wounded when we were imprinted in this way. The generation before us was not aware of these dynamics. We adapted as they did and lost contact with our "double" like they often did. This is how the cycle has repeated itself through the generations. For our children to make contact with their real selves in adolescence, we must individuate in midlife.

If we do not heed the call to live authentically, we risk living from our adaptations and *pretending* to be real. The symptoms of this are pervasive in our society. Overconsumption is a compensated behavior that we engage in due to our disconnection from what is real. We over-consume in order to compensate for our feelings of emptiness. We may be unaware of this until our forties. At this juncture, the changes in our hormones uncover and unleash the unindividuated and unprocessed parts of our psyches through our feeling function in order to make them conscious. Feelings of anger and sadness may surface. This can be confusing for many. Our bodies mark this powerful time of cleansing when it becomes necessary to release the life patterns that cause our suffering.

The depth of the midlife process

For women, this time is usually marked by hormonal changes which unleash a torrent of emotions and intense feelings that can often be overwhelming. Many women feel like they are "going crazy" as their hormones begin to change.

In my own life, I felt a rustling inside that indicated that my life as I knew it would be coming to an end. I was 42 and had been in an unhealthy relationship. I was unable to leave it due to my imprinted and conditioned patterns. A few years after this feeling surfaced, my life, as I knew it, was blown to pieces.

This was an intense process that flooded me with deep feelings of grief and loss. I was being asked to reconfigure my thinking from the inside out. I was betrayed in a relationship that I held sacred even after years of abuse. My conditioning directed me to adapt to the abuse. I unknowingly allowed this, as many of us do. Sometimes we adapt by growing numb to the pain of being disrespected and dishonored. Through our adaptations, we become desensitized to escalating pain in order to "keep the peace." This process is called *learned help-lessness*. If the system we live in feels familiar, we are fearful to leave it. The pain we imagine from losing the relationship may feel worse than the pain of the abuse within it. Fear distorts our perceptions and we becoming willing to adapt to abuse because of it. Sometimes the abuse is emotional and sometimes it is physical. Sometimes it is both. Emotional abuse is often harder to acknowledge as it does not leave physical scars, but is just as damaging as physical abuse. Often it is harder to leave relationships that are emotionally abusive due to our adaptations. If we are unable to leave a relationship that causes us pain, it has deeply disempowered us. These are the effects of living in a closed system. Sometimes, when abuse and pain escalate to a great degree, the system ruptures. Betrayal ruptured mine. I was unwilling to adapt to this level of disrespect.

It was my time to sort through the rubble that contained my adapted and conditioned parts and reexamine who I really was. I needed to individuate from my adapted self, and intrinsically reinvent myself. I began to consciously dismantle all of the parts of me that resulted from my familial imprinting that I had mistakenly identified as my real self. I offered myself choices between who I thought I was and what felt true to my authentic and real self. I was making contact with my "double." Wholeness had beckoned, and I chose to step in.

As terrified as I was to leave the abusive relationship, to my surprise, its rupture unraveled a process that felt richer and more meaningful in many ways than anything I had experienced before. The gates of hell had opened, and with intense fear and great courage, I fell into the abyss. In that moment of pure anguish, my "double" spoke to me with a deep inner voice that I recognized as my own. I felt that my life would be reborn from the bottom of the abyss. It was.

I surrendered my tired and broken self that could no longer adapt and fell into the abyss with profound grief and despair. The deep shock of betrayal dismantled my adapted life. Despite false voices from the culture that told me to "get over it," I chose to feel every feeling to its true depth. This was the way my wounded instinct and my feeling function would heal while I reconnected with the voice of my soul and my real self. As I continued to heed this voice, I grew stronger and my instinct was able to guide me in directions that I would have never considered before.

Synchronicities began to occur in my life, and I felt as if I were embarking on a higher destiny directed by my soul. It felt unfamiliar than the one that I had lived from before. My "double" had charted a course correction and directed me back on a path that my true self had always been seeking. I was healing after four decades of being wounded. I began to trust in my process and heal the fear of being true to myself. My instinct and feeling function became key elements of my inner guidance from that moment forward.

My intense love for my children was a constant source of strength through this process. My commitment to them held the deepest meaning and offered me the greatest courage to move along this difficult path when I felt tired and hopeless. In those moments, I had to take responsibility for my role in the wreckage that had occurred in *their* lives as a result of my disconnection from my real self. Although I was unaware of this disconnection as an unindividuated woman and felt profound loneliness because of it, I realized that the opportunity to create an authentic life lay before me that could provide mentorship and support for them. I also needed to forgive myself for remaining unconscious and adapted for so long.

This was an intense process. I watched my children trying to adapt to the rupture of our family by normalizing and adapting in order to survive. I struggled with an almost other-worldly grief. I had repressed my feeling function for years in order to survive in a relationship that required me to deny my truth and sovereignty. I learned to often project a mask of "happiness" that others expected to see. My grief decimated this mask. My feeling function required me to connect with my feelings of outrage that I was expected to suppress. I needed to bring who I really was into alignment with my feeling function. This process was profoundly difficult and profoundly healing. Through it, I found myself connected with women all over the world who were also reclaiming their truth and sovereignty. In addition, I found myself connected with my ancestors, women who had gone before me, who capitulated to society's expectations of being "a good wife" and tolerated abuse as a mark of "a strong woman." It was as though my feeling function, lying dormant for generations had resurrected, and I was given the opportunity to use the alchemical qualities of my soul to make something of worth and meaning from my pain.

I had to redefine all of the ways that I had perceived reality. I had to learn how to first connect with, and then validate and honor my feeling function which I was told for the first half of my life was "wrong," was "too intense" and was a threat to the status quo.

I realized that my definitions of love, power, truth and worth needed to be continually re-evaluated. I needed to purify them through what felt true for *me*. The definitions from society felt superficial and distorted. They fostered codependency and made me vulnerable to the type of abuse that I had experienced. I recognized that the wisdom in my feeling function was able to discern what felt healthy and what didn't. It was resurrecting itself after half a lifetime of being wounded. This would help me recreate my life from a place of *my* truth. I needed to trust that my truth and feelings were "right."

This process was painful and intensely difficult. I lived in constant fear of being rejected by others, of being left alone in a world that normalized dishonesty, adultery, misogyny and adapted behaviors. My perception of the world began to change and I realized that the world itself needed guidance in these areas. I felt that I could play a part in healing our culture's collective and unhealthy patterns. My alchemical process catalyzed these insights. My midlife patients were doing this work in their own lives, and I was part of a community of courageous transformation. I realized that this was the important work of our generation. We needed to individuate in order to collectively transform adapted patterns that were normalized yet unhealthy and unfulfilling. This could bring powerful and precise meaning to our suffering. If I could consciously individuate through my midlife gateway, and recreate myself through mentorship from my "double," I could earn the ability to mentor my children and future generations from a place that was real. I knew that I needed to live from my truth from that moment forward and behave in ways that honored my feeling function and my instinct.

I realized that this was an important part of my work as a woman, a mother, an Indian, an American and also a physician. I was being called by my higher destiny to help dismantle the unhealthy and adapted patterns that I had normalized that allowed me to be treated with dishonor and redefine Women's Health through this deeper place that honored the Feminine Principle.

The midlife process in health care

As my perspective deepened, I was able to see more clearly how women were frequently dismissed by the health care system if they sought solutions to their common midlife symptoms. If their feeling function was heightened and they expressed it, they were often considered pathological and medicated. They frequently had no voice to speak their truth. What they needed was for physicians to bear witness to their biographies and their stories. Through the limited lens of the current health care system, they felt unsafe in their own skins and frightened by their feelings.

I realized that women were looking for something more than what the current health care system offered. Women's Health, defined by that system was too limited, too physical, too physiological and too superficial. Women's stories and feelings had no place in it. These aspects of their lives were integral to their journeys towards health. These stories held powerful "medicine" for them to connect with their real selves. The limited space that their physicians held did not facilitate their transformation. Women needed a framework that could mirror for them their greatness and their highest potential so they could connect with their truth. They needed to be received in a sacred space where they could feel safe enough to honestly reckon with who they had become as adapted and wounded women, and confront the shame that this evoked. They needed a place where they could feel unconditionally supported through their midlife process.

Shame is the toxic feeling that contaminates a woman's relationship towards herself. She feels it when she views herself through her critical lens, or when she behaves in ways that compromise her truth. Shame is always a sign that a woman's shadow is near. Women in midlife want to purify their relationships to themselves by living from integrity and truth despite the lives they may have created from their adaptations and conditioned behaviors. Sometimes shame can serve as a catalyst to transform these adapted patterns. It can be the feeling that awakens women to the inauthentic relationships that they may have had with themselves. In midlife, they can no longer lie to themselves and pretend that their façades are real.

Women live with shame for most of their lives. For many, it is loud and looming. It manifests in avoidant behaviors that can isolate them from others. It often compromises their ability to speak their truth. It is based in fear. It makes them vulnerable in relationships that operate from the dynamics of closed systems. These behaviors are unfulfilling. We feel shame when we compromise ourselves through our adapted behaviors but we also feel it when we attempt to live from our truth and disappoint others. In the former situation, we feel shame due to self-betrayal; in the latter, shame is inflicted upon us by others for not normalizing their unhealthy dynamics. It can be confusing to differentiate between these feelings of shame. Either one can drive us to behave in compensated ways and self-medicate. These compensating behaviors deplete us and often make us ill. We need to remember that the shame we feel due to self-betrayal can serve as a healthy signal that reminds us to live from our truth; the other kind of shame is unhealthy and needs to be processed and released. Many women long for a safe space where their recovery from shame can be held as a sacred process, while they orient themselves back to their truth.

When I work with women, the festering wounds caused by shame are often exposed. When I ask crucial questions and bring integrity and truth to the space I hold, they are able to confront their shame and heal it. Women often gain the ability to identify the many faces of shame that exist in their psyches. They gain the needed awareness that can prevent them from behaving in compensated ways that betray their truth. It is difficult to awaken to this in isolation. We often need others to bring this to consciousness for us to heal these patterns.

In order to safely facilitate another's movement toward what is real, we must first engage in our own personal work of individuation. We cannot help others arrive at a place that we have not arrived at ourselves. Our physician and therapist offices are filled with wounded practitioners, those who are not individuated, and haven't had the courage to do the real work of their own transformation. They are unable to help others fully transform as they themselves lack the insight needed to help others navigate through territories that lead to the connection with what is real. In fact, being held in this kind of space can be dangerous for a patient's difficult and confusing process. The practitioner's ignorance can subvert their patient's transformation. They are unable to take their clients to a place beyond their own levels of growth. We need to bring an understanding of this crucial element of process to our professional and cultural framework, and guide each other through the treacherous territories of individuation with clarity and integrity. This requires us to stand in the fire of our own transformation and identify with our real selves so we can safely guide others to connect with what is real for them.

What had awakened in me through my own midlife process was deeper and more powerful than anything I could have imagined. I always felt that there was more to the medical model than what I had been taught. I had felt profound loneliness during my medical training since I did not resonate with the limited lens through which I was taught to evaluate and treat patients. This lens did not include the possibility for patients to heal their lives or live from their greatness. I realized how I had suffered as a result of this limited perspective which led to feelings of powerlessness in my own life. Having gone through my own transformation enabled me to hold space for women who were seeking to transform in my care.

An authentic medical practice

When I realized that I shared in this collective wound, I knew that I needed to do my part in shedding light on it in order to understand it and heal.

In my own process as I grieved the loss of all that I held sacred, I connected with my ability to create my higher destiny. I also confronted my fear of being rejected from my family and society when I redefined myself in unfamiliar and healthy ways. At this point, I had nothing to lose. If I were "loved" as a reward for being obedient to familial and cultural definitions, then this love was not real. It was a distortion. It was a conditioned reward for my obedience to a construct that kept the closed system's shadow hidden. As I transformed into my authentic self, I was able to reconnect with my family from a healthier place without compromising my truth.

"Getting over" our feelings

We are often told to "get over" how we feel if our feelings carry depth or intensity. Many in our culture are not comfortable around strong feelings. We have to honor our feelings and *not* take in these injunctions. We need to examine what it means to "get over" feelings. Does it mean that we are expected to deny our feeling function and subdue our truth in order to perpetuate the status quo of the closed system? In my case, many around me expected me to "get over" my grief and anger towards how I had been treated. This injunction challenged my process that was attempting to connect me with my real self. I could not obey these injunctions and expect to connect with my intrinsic power. Furthermore, I had a responsibility to my children to be true to myself. They had witnessed the ways I had adapted to abuse and who I had become in an unhealthy relationship. I could not mentor them effectively or honestly if I obeyed these injunctions and continued to betray myself. This would perpetuate my façade of "happiness." I could no longer live from that adapted place.

As I questioned this injunction and refused to obey it, I began to find my voice which connected me to my deep feeling function. We often apologize for our feeling function when it seeps through our tears as we attempt to speak our truth. When we subdue our feeling function, it manifests as the neuroses that keep us awake at night. We try to "keep the peace" in order to not "rock the boat," but our feelings arises in midlife in ways that are intense and powerful. Our feelings are the voices of our intuition, our instincts and the means through which our inner wisdom communicates. We must stop apologizing for them.

As I disobeyed the injunctions to "get over" my feelings and practiced becoming comfortable with my strong feeling function, I made a conscious commitment to myself. I vowed that I would never compromise my feelings in obedience to society's expectations. These expectations were society's attempts to perpetuate its closed systems.

This wisdom gave me both the strength and courage to empower other women to do the same. This was the beginning of both a personal transformation and a collective awakening within my medical practice. I was "coming into my own." I was individuating.

Healthy love as unfamiliar

A few years after I made this commitment to myself, love reappeared in my life. But this time it was an unfamiliar love that felt uncontaminated and healthy. I believe that my connection to my truth magnetized it. I was willing to be alone for the rest of my life if living from my truth was not acceptable to others. This love emerged as a result of the undistorted definitions that I was beginning to live from. It was strong enough to accept me for who I authentically was. It held space for my process and expected no compromise of my real self. Even though I had never experienced this before and did not have a relative position to define this, it felt healthy. Previously, I was expected to sacrifice myself in order to "hold it together" while compromising my truth and my power. I was driven by my conditioning to keep it together at all costs.

I realized that my "double" had laid out a path for my individuating self to experience the uncontaminated definitions of love, power and worth. She was supporting the choices that I was making from a place of courage and truth, and no longer from fear.

A healthy relationship in midlife is one that supports and strengthens our sovereignty and our movement toward wholeness. It can support the call from the "double" and mirror Her back to us when we forget to live from Her direction and guidance. A healthy relationship may feel unfamiliar, but it can be seen as a powerful sign for the reclamation of our health. Unhealthy relationships before the midlife gateway can also be transformed into healthy ones through engaging both the consciousness and courage that is required to uncover our authenticity and truth.

The juncture point in midlife

At the end of our lives, before the final gateway of death, we are guaranteed a life review when we will have to come to terms with the choices we made from either fear or courage. Like Alice, any fear-based choices that took us off course will cause us great anxiety. We all hope to die with peace in our hearts. In order for us to die in peace, we must connect with our real selves in midlife and live from our higher destinies for the second half of our lives. Serving the expectations of the world will not bring us any peace.

The process of individuation, is one in which the precision in life reveals itself. This precision brings us into contact with the sacred. When seen through this perspective, our life's purpose can be revealed through recovery from our previously adapted lives. When we become real, we can guide others with what we have learned. This process is alchemical and is often catalyzed by pain. We must feel our feelings fully and deeply in order for them to completely transform us. Choosing health after being adapted can feel confusing and unfamiliar. Our choices may feel counterintuitive, but they can heal our wounded instincts and make our inner truth and wisdom more accessible. They can correct the course of our lives. They can also offer us much needed solace at the end of our lives when we can feel comforted for having lived from a place of authenticity and integrity.

For midlife women, in their late thirties, changes in their bodies begin subtly, hinting of hormonal imbalance before their periods as their feeling function heightens. They may suddenly find themselves unable to tolerate the ways in which they have adapted to the expectations of the world. During their forties, this process intensifies. Hormonal shifts widen, changing biology and uncovering the previously repressed details of biography, bringing them into consciousness for review and deconstruction of familial patterns. Individuation beckons with deep intensity and sometimes fury.

I became fascinated by the power with which hormonal changes unleashed intense feelings and alchemical energy in women. I observed this as part of my own transformation as my early morning awakenings were wrought with fear and then followed by intense creativity. This process was deeply personal and I moved through it alone. As my adapted life was falling to pieces, my "double" was unfolding my true destiny. I was learning Her language through my feelings, night after night. I began to furiously journal, weaving my patients' similar stories through the framework I was learning from this deeper part of me. All parts of my life revealed a precision that I saw for the first time. As I applied this framework to my patients' lives, they were able to see their wholeness through it and became empowered. Women began to leave the victimized place from which they had been living. Their pain and wounding began to make sense and they were able to use them as catalysts to uncover the parts of themselves that they needed to cultivate and reclaim. They were able to see the wisdom in the chaos that they had frequently felt as they recognized the sacred theme their lives held that reverberated through their life experiences. They realized that if they reframed their perspective, they could release the illusion of their smallness and make contact with the unlimited potential contained within their real selves. They could mobilize their awareness and reframe their roles as heroines in their biographies rather than victims. They could use the inner pressure that was caused by their suppressed feelings alchemically, and transform into their authentic and real selves. This connected them to their truth and wisdom. They gained access to their potential to activate their intrinsic power and with that, their presence and reclaim the joy that had been missing in their lives.

Our body as the initiator

During childhood, our bodies initiate us through menses from children into maidens. They initiate many through pregnancy into motherhood. Our bodies also connect us with a deeper sense of meaning through illness.

Menopause is our body's way of initiating us yet again. First, towards the end of our thirties, our feelings begin to intensify. Next, in our forties, our emotions escalate with gusto and added physical symptoms. Our "double" begins to call to us through our bodies due to the parting of our hormonal seas. As our progesterone level falls, it creates biological imbalance that calls for the restoration of balance, and our lost self calls for a connection to what is real. We begin to hear the voice of our "double" through the intensity of our feelings. She asks us to make choices that can help us to connect with our real selves. She offers us the door to the unknown that is frightening and unfamiliar yet leads to our higher destiny. This is the other door, the door that Alice did not walk through, despite promptings from her "double." This is the door we must walk through in order to live from our real selves.

It is a great honor and privilege to work with this transformative midlife initiation. The sacred is acutely palpable in this gateway when the veil between the conscious and unconscious self grows thin. This is where the soul seeps through. The soul speaks through their feelings and dreams of the courageous people who are consciously journeying through this portal in order to connect with their real selves. They are often awed by their new found level of self-worth and capability. Fear is replaced by trust in the process. As they upgrade their choices, they begin to emit an energy that is intensely beautiful in this initiatory state. They can finally connect to their inner greatness—a place within that they may have never felt before. They begin behaving as though they embody their holy "double." They begin living from a place of curiosity and wonder, and are able to utilize the discernment they have gained for over half a lifetime in order to live from their inner wisdom that they now can access.

The biological changes women go through in midlife are powerful and fascinating. The fact that they evoke deeper levels of transformation is a framework that is necessary for us to incorporate in order for Women's Health to be effective. Sadly, what physicians have done thus far has been to prescribe medications and dismiss the symptoms of transformation and rising feeling function during menopause as pathological rather than alchemical and powerful.

We need to reframe menopause as a sacred initiation. Currently, we need to redefine leadership in our society as one that integrates the elements of the Feminine Principle. Our institutions of medicine, finance, politics, religion and education all suffer from the lack of the healthy feminine. Our sacred work as midlife women is to awaken to our truth, and reclaim it until we feel comfortable in our new skins. Only after undergoing this process, can we bring our real selves through our actions, behaviors and presence into the world, and transform its illness into health.

We also need to understand our bodies so as to not fear the changes that this midlife transition brings. What we do not understand makes us fearful. As a health care provider, it is my responsibility and vocation to educate and reframe the symptoms that menopause elicits in order to help women understand them as signals of transformation. This framework has the ability to dispel the fear of this transition, by uncovering the power and precision of our biology. It is essential for us to mark our initiatory passages which have been neglected and dismissed by our culture and the current medical system. Many women feel lost and alone, struggling through their transition with no guidance, wishing they could turn back their biological clocks and become young again.

It is important and critical for our health, to balance all levels of the body. We must always remember that this medial time in midlife is one of great power that calls us to reframe our definitions of meaning and health. Success can no longer be defined by society's standards, but from the inner place that is restless and no longer fulfilled by material and superficial trappings. Our authentic "double" calls us to go within and speaks to us through our restless nights and our feelings of longing. We are called to deconstruct our old adapted selves and are presented with opportunities and choices through our midlife gateways to individuate from familiar patterns that have deprived us of meaning in order to evoke the beauty of what is real and authentic for us.

The holy "double" never rests. Her language is one of "rest-lest-ness." This may manifest as feelings of anxiety, depression and loneliness when we do not connect to Her. When we obey Her call and ask crucial questions like "why are we here, how can we live authentically and how can we die a good death," She settles and grants us a good night's sleep. Our depression and anxiety heal and life takes on a deeper level of meaning. We must ask these crucial questions during our midlife gateway. Our answers to them and the choices we make will help us unfold the second half of our lives. We must remember that we have deep inner guidance, the voice of restlessness within that keeps us loyal company and only settles when we live out the important answers and unfold our higher destinies.

Every woman's journey is unique and sacred. It is deeply influenced by her biography, her heritage and her environment. To be able to weave these together and gain understanding from this sacred perspective is critical for our connection with our souls' purpose. The midlife gateway marked by menopause, carries within it the potential to transform us into our real and authentic selves. Moving through this process with consciousness holds the keys to our future joy and fulfillment.

Becoming real is necessary and urgent in our world today. We must keep this intention close to our hearts. If we answer the call from our "double" and transform, we will never feel lost or alone again.

3

The Female Body in Midlife

Carla

Carla is a 48-year-old woman who came to me to find relief from her perimenopausal symptoms. I asked her about her understanding of the menstrual cycle. She began to weep, ashamed of her ignorance. For thirty-five years, she had not understood her monthly cycles. She was thirteen when she began menses and every month, she looked forward to the day she would stop bleeding. Menses felt like an illness and a nuisance to her as her premenstrual symptoms were intense. She did not understand the biological or symbolic meaning of her cycles, and none of her physicians had explained them to her. As her mother had not understood this herself, she also had been unable to educate Carla. Now, Carla was in the perimenopausal transition experiencing symptoms of emotional agitation, headaches, insomnia and hot flashes. As I explained this process to her, Carla was relieved. She was never taught how to honor it as one of great power. With an understanding from this deeper perspective, she felt both a sense of relief and loss. For most of her life, she had missed the opportunity to connect with her cycles from a sacred perspective.

It caused me sadness to bear witness to Carla's grief. Despite the information available today, many women are uninformed about the biology and meaning of their menstrual cycles. It is important for us to have an understanding of our cycles in order to effectively care for ourselves. This may seem intimidating for many, but for as long as we remain ignorant, we remain fearful. With an understanding of our biology, we can make sense of our symptoms and their biological causes, and can consciously care for ourselves during menses and menopause. Without this understanding, there is danger for us to remain disempowered and dependent upon medical experts who are more focused on symptom management than on healing or wholeness.

Female hormones

The female ovary produces three main hormones:
1. Estrogen
2. Progesterone
3. Testosterone

Estrogen
Stated simply, estrogen is the hormone that both females and males produce, but females produce it in greater quantities.

Estrogen:
- is responsible for the development of breasts, uterine tissue and vaginal wall thickness
- has effects on multiple other organ systems, including the liver and the digestive system where it decreases motility and increases absorption of nutrients
- affects bone density, where it decreases breakdown or turnover of bone

Estrone, Estradiol and Estriol are the three main estrogens made in the human body. These are referred to in science as E1, E2 and E3.
- **Estrone (E1)** is produced in the ovary and in large percentage by fat cells. It is the least abundant of the three estrogenic hormones. It is the primary estrogen produced during menopause, but in small amounts.

- **Estradiol (E2)** is produced by the ovaries and is the estrogen responsible for the female cycles and development of sexual characteristics. It is the culprit in many breast cancers, breast cysts, fibroadenomas, endometriosis and fibroid tumors. When levels begin to decline in the fourth decade of life, symptoms of perimenopause such as hot flashes and night sweats can become prevalent.

- **Estriol (E3)** is a form of estrogen that is produced almost exclusively during pregnancy by the developing fetus. It crosses the placental barrier and enters the mother's body during pregnancy. Estriol is mostly responsible for the integrity of the vagina, cervix and vulva. It has little to no impact on breast or uterine tissue.

Progesterone

Progesterone is a hormone produced by the ovaries and the adrenal glands and also during pregnancy by the placenta. Its main role is to maintain the lining of the uterus after ovulation so the fertilized egg can implant onto this lining to develop into a baby. Progesterone has profound effects on many other areas of a woman's body.

Progesterone:
- effects mood by increasing the level of serotonin
- promotes muscle relaxation
- stimulates bone growth
- stimulates nerve growth
- promotes healthy skin and hair
- assists in thyroid balance
- has anti-inflammatory properties
- decreases tissue and muscle stiffness, and hence muscle injury
- decreases heavy menstrual flow
- effects the tone of the urinary sphincter, the urethra. A decrease in its level can cause urinary leakage.
- regulates the sleep cycle
- relaxes the digestive system and affects the motility (movement) of the gut and the intestine

- acts as a diuretic (decreases water retention)
- counterbalances the effects of estrogen
- lowers blood pressure
- decreases coronary spasm

An imbalance between estrogen and progesterone, where the estrogen level is high and not counterbalanced by adequate levels of progesterone can cause premenstrual syndrome (PMS) and a myriad of perimenopausal symptoms. The balance of estrogen and progesterone is also protective against breast cancer, breast and ovarian cysts, fibroid tumor formation, and endometriosis.

Progesterone balance is so important that if its level remains low relative to estrogen, resulting in a high estrogen to progesterone ratio, women can be more prone to breast and uterine cancers, strokes, hypertension and heart attacks. These diseases are prevalent in epidemic proportions in the Western Hemisphere.

Testosterone

Testosterone is produced in women in small amounts in the ovaries and the adrenal glands.

Testosterone:
- is responsible for a woman's sex drive
- affects feelings of vitality and energy
- affects the potency of a woman's orgasm and sensitivity of her erogenous zones
- increases muscle tone and muscle mass
- to a small degree, increases tone of the urinary sphincter

When the ovaries begin to wind down in a woman's late thirties and forties, the testosterone level begins to fall. Women may feel a decrease in libido and vitality and may also experience urinary leakage and irritation of the urinary sphincter due to the fall in this level.

DHEA

DHEA (dehydroepiandrosterone) is a hormone that is produced by the adrenal glands and is a precursor of female and male reproductive hormones (estrogen, progesterone and androgens). *A precursor is a cellular substance or protein from which other proteins and hormones are made.* When a woman has adrenal fatigue, her DHEA level can decline. The DHEA level naturally decreases after the third decade of life. If the level decreases too much, this can sometimes indicate adrenal fatigue.

The menstrual cycle

The menstrual cycle can be understood in simple terms that demystify what we have often felt to be a complex biological process. Any time between the approximate ages of ten and thirteen, a girl's pituitary gland (*an endocrine gland in the brain that regulates hormone production*) begins to produce two hormones, Follicle Stimulating Hormone or FSH and Luteinizing Hormone or LH.

- FSH stimulates a part of the ovary called the follicle to produce estrogen. The *follicular phase* of the menstrual cycle is the phase between menses and ovulation, from days 0 to 14 (figure 1). During this phase, the egg grows and develops under the influence of estrogen, in order to prepare it for ovulation, when it is released from the ovary in anticipation for its potential fertilization by a sperm. Estrogen causes the lining of the uterus to build for potential implantation of the fertilized egg.

- LH stimulates ovulation together with FSH around day twelve to fourteen, in the middle of the cycle, when there is an abrupt increase in both FSH as well as LH levels. It marks the beginning of the *luteal phase* (days 14 to 28). Menses often begins on day 28 of the cycle.

As soon as ovulation occurs, the egg is released from the ovary and journeys to the uterus for its potential fertilization by a sperm. The corpus luteum, or sac, that housed the egg inside the ovary begins to produce progesterone.

Progesterone protects the uterus from shedding its lining that estrogen carefully created in the *follicular phase* so that the fertilized egg can implant within it and grow into a baby. If the egg is not fertilized, the progesterone level begins to drop by day 24 and approximately fourteen days after ovulation the uterine lining is shed with an abrupt fall in progesterone (figure 1). This is referred to as menstruation or menses.

The time between ovulation and menses is called the *luteal phase* of the menstrual cycle, when the corpus luteum produces progesterone. This is sometimes the most emotionally difficult time of the menstrual cycle for women who do not ovulate regularly or do not produce enough progesterone upon ovulation. Progesterone intricately impacts a woman's emotional health and well-being. The balance or imbalance between the estrogen and progesterone level

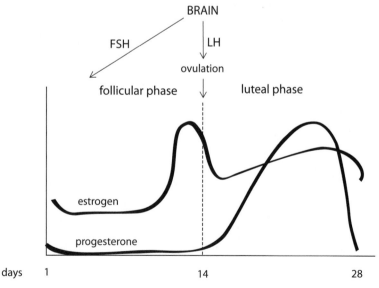

Figure 1: The female menstrual cycle

is what is felt in the Emotional body. Often in their late thirties, women begin to skip ovulation, and their progesterone level drops, creating an imbalance in the estrogen to progesterone ratio. This results in estrogen becoming the more "dominant" hormone when the progesterone level falls. This imbalance is termed "estrogen dominance." This is one of the main causes for premenstrual and perimenopausal symptoms.

Estrogen dominance

In the U.S., estrogen dominance occurs in epidemic proportions as compared to other countries. Our foods are contaminated with synthetic estrogens, or *xenoestrogens* from many different sources. One source is the synthetic hormones that are fed to animals to increase their yield of meat and dairy. When we consume these animals, the fed hormones become concentrated in our bodies. This occurs when humans consume any pesticides, medications or hormones that animals are fed. Both pesticides and hormones become more concentrated as they move up the food chain and into the human body. For example, if a plant eaten by an animal is sprayed with a pesticide, it becomes more concentrated in the animal. If the animal is then given synthetic hormones to increase its yield and humans eat this animal, the humans get a more concentrated load of pesticides in addition to the hormones that the animal receives. Xenoestrogens are one of the breakdown products of the many of the pesticides used to spray crops in the U.S. They are also the breakdown products from plastics. Synthetic hormones prescribed by the medical system as HRT or Hormone Replacement Therapy are a source of synthetic estrogens. Synthetic estrogens over-stimulate the estrogen receptors present on the surface of cells, and accentuate symptoms of estrogen dominance in humans. *A receptor is the part on the cell surface that the hormone or protein binds to, causing a reaction inside the cell.*

In other countries, estrogen to progesterone imbalance or estrogen dominance is not as significant due to lower to no levels of xenoestrogens contained in foods and the higher consumption of soy and plant-based foods. Soy contains phytoestrogens or plant based estrogens that protect the estrogen receptor from overstimulation by xeno or synthetic estrogens. Estrogen dominance is more prevalent in women in the U.S. due to the quantity of synthetic hormones prescribed and the elevated xenoestrogen load in the foods consumed in the U.S.

Stress is an important factor that contributes to the imbalance in the estrogen to progesterone ratio. Stress hormones lower the progesterone level. Much stress is caused by the lack of support we feel from the loss of our connection to each other. Less than thirty years ago, people were valued as a part of their community or village. This provided them with an emotional buffer for life's stressors. Since we no longer have this level of support, we deal with stress alone. This causes significant increases in stress hormones produced by the adrenal glands. It puts us in a frequent state of survival. This survival state triggers the "the fight-or-flight" response. The body reacts to stress by getting ready to either fight or flee. This causes the production of high levels of adrenalin, the most common stress hormone produced by the adrenal glands. Sometimes, under conditions of chronic stress, survival can become a chronic state of living which triggers the adrenals glands to produce high levels the stress hormone, cortisol. (The adrenal glands also produce other hormones that benefit our health and regulate our bodily functions). When too much cortisol is produced under conditions of chronic stress, it can cause unhealthy effects on the body. Some of these are:

- weight gain
- depression
- fatigue
- increase in stomach acid

- increase in cholesterol
- increase in blood sugar
- increase in appetite
- increase in blood pressure or hypertension
- spasm of the coronary arteries (the arteries that supply the heart with oxygenated blood)
- decrease in memory
- thinning of skin and hair
- suppression of the immune system

There are two factors that reduce progesterone levels when women are under conditions of chronic stress.

1. Cortisol competes with progesterone for the ability to bind to its receptors on the surface of the cell. This accelerates a decline in the amount of progesterone that can enter the cell to create health and balance. This decline in the progesterone level exaggerates the estrogen to progesterone imbalance and contributes to estrogen dominance.

2. Cortisol suppresses the *production* of progesterone. When cortisol levels rise due to stress, progesterone levels often decrease. Both of these factors lead to reduction in progesterone levels relative to estrogen, contributing to estrogen dominance.

Women who are emotionally sensitive tend to produce higher concentrations of stress hormones while under stress. Since they feel deeply, they also feel stress more intensely. Because of their increased sensitivity, they can also feel restorations in balance with natural hormones more rapidly.

Hormone testing

Hormone levels can be tested in blood or saliva. In the past twenty years of medical practice, I have found that blood levels offer a more accurate correlation to a woman's symptoms. Many medical practices utilize the latter as their favored test. In my experience, the saliva test is cumbersome and expensive and carries a high percentage of procedural error. The accuracy of saliva testing is unknown when saliva samples are shipped in extreme weather conditions without the proper packaging needed to maintain the integrity of this secretion. When hormone levels are measured simultaneously with blood, the blood levels appear to more accurately correlate with how a woman feels. This is helpful in adjusting the doses of natural hormones prescribed. It helps ensure her from being over or under medicated and is more likely to assure hormone balance.

Depending upon a woman's stage of menopause, an estrogen to progesterone ratio (estrogen/progesterone) of *two to ten*, measured in the blood, seems to be the ideal ratio for achieving hormone balance. Perimenopausal women tend to feel better with an estrogen to progesterone ratio of *six to ten*, and menopausal women with a ratio of *two to five*. These are approximate estimates and should be monitored by a physician who is skilled in natural hormone balance. The levels should always be correlated to symptomatic relief or clinical response that a woman experiences. The goal of balance is to use the *least* amount of hormone for the *greatest* clinical benefit. *Balance*, not replacement, should be the goal of prescribing natural hormones. Balancing hormones is as much an art as it is a science.

Estrogen or Estradiol (E2)

Estradiol (E2) is the form of estrogen that is most frequently measured. This is the estrogen that needs to be balanced with progesterone. Estradiol levels can be measured through a blood test. Its levels when measured during days 21 to 24 of the menstrual cycle with progesterone, can offer a fairly accurate reading of a woman's state of hormone balance. If the estradiol level is too high, and a woman is taking natural estrogen, the dose of natural estrogen should be decreased. If a woman is not taking natural estrogen, but is on natural progesterone, and blood levels reflect an estrogen dominance pattern, the physician must decrease the dose of progesterone as the cause of the high estrogen level can be due to progesterone's conversion to estrogen. Progesterone's timing of use in the menstrual cycle should then be carefully assessed. If it is administered during the follicular phase, it has a greater probability of conversion to estrogen.

Progesterone

Progesterone has a slight estrogenic effect that can abate some of the common symptoms of estrogen withdrawal such as hot flashes and night sweats that are caused by the decreased production of ovarian estradiol. Hormone levels need to be measured periodically if a woman is taking natural progesterone, due to the possibility its conversion to estrogen. A clinical sign of progesterone to estrogen conversion would be the aggravation of symptoms of estrogen dominance. If a perimenopausal woman takes natural progesterone during the *follicular phase* of her cycle (day 0 to 14), she has a greater probability of converting the progesterone into estrogen due to the estrogenic influence of the body during this phase of the cycle. In other words, when the body is geared towards producing estrogen during the *follicular phase* of the menstrual cycle, it is more likely to convert progesterone into estrogen during this phase. Natural progesterone taken during the *luteal phase* is less likely to be converted to estrogen.

It is important to measure estrogen and progesterone levels every 3 months until a woman's levels become balanced and stay consistent. The best time to measure estrogen and progesterone levels to assess balance is during days 21 to 24 of the menstrual cycle. This gives the most accurate reading for a state of balance. In menopausal women (who are not menstruating), hormone levels can be measured at any time of the month as they no longer cycle.

Testosterone

Free testosterone is testosterone that is freely available to affect the body. *Total* testosterone is the combination of levels of *free* testosterone and testosterone bound to albumin (*a kind of protein*). *Free* testosterone levels give a measure of the testosterone level in a woman's body that is actively working. Free testosterone levels can be measured by a blood test to determine if a woman needs supplementation with natural testosterone for symptoms caused by low testosterone.

Free and *total* testosterone levels can be measured in the blood if a woman has symptoms of a decreasing libido and vitality. If her *free* testosterone level is low, her physician can prescribe natural testosterone in the form of a cream, gel or capsule. If a woman experiences chronic urinary tract infections after menopause, she can also benefit from the application of natural testosterone to the urinary (urethral) opening and vulva as it can reduce the incidence of these infections.

It is important to check *free* testosterone levels at least every three months after beginning natural testosterone treatment because its level can rapidly increase causing acne, facial hair, emotional irritability and *conversion to estrogen.* Testosterone can also be converted into estrogen, particularly after menopause through a reaction that occurs in the cells. This can aggravate estrogen dominance, so it is important to manage the prescribed dose with blood levels under the guidance of a physician. Initially, a woman may benefit from daily natural testosterone usage, but once a therapeutic level is reached, she may not need to take the full dose on a daily basis.

The risks of estrogen dominance

A worrisome fact about women in the U.S. compared to women in other countries is the high concentrations of estrogen present in their body fat.

This is due to two factors:

1. High concentrations of synthetic estrogens present in food in the U.S. through widespread use of pesticides and synthetic hormones by "agribusiness."

2. Moderate use of synthetic hormones ingested by women in the form of oral contraceptives and hormone replacement therapies.

Farming practices in the U.S., where pesticides and synthetic hormones are used, have high concentrations of xenoestrogens in the animal runoff from farms. In addition, women using oral contraceptives and synthetic hormone replacement therapy excrete moderate amounts of synthetic hormone fragments in their urine which filters down into the groundwater. This increases the groundwater concentration of synthetic estrogens. When we drink the water containing synthetic estrogens, it is more likely to accumulate in our bodies causing estrogen dominance.

Estrogen dominance makes us vulnerable to the diseases that are caused by estrogen excess. Some of these diseases are:

- breast cancer
- uterine cancer
- fibroids
- endometriosis
- fibrocystic breasts
- insulin resistance
- increase in blood cholesterol levels
- strokes
- hypertension
- blood clots
- obesity
- infertility
- coronary artery spasm resulting in increased risk of heart attacks

- suppression of the immune system
- urinary leakage

Some symptoms of estrogen dominance are:

- heavy periods
- intermittent bleeding during the menstrual cycle
- mood swings
- breast tenderness
- headaches
- water retention
- fatigue
- foggy thinking
- decrease in memory
- abdominal bloating
- irritable bowel symptoms such as constipation and diarrhea
- dry skin
- insomnia
- accelerated signs of aging
- muscle pain
- mild vertigo
- thinning of hair

Many of these symptoms can also be experienced with declining progesterone levels. Without adequate blood levels of progesterone, we are more vulnerable to these conditions as we grow older. We feel them with greater vigor in our forties when progesterone levels decline and the imbalance between estrogen and progesterone is more pronounced. They become less pronounced after menopause as both hormone levels decline. At this time, small doses of progesterone are protective and can also help symptoms of estrogen withdrawal (such as hot flashes and night sweats). Estrogen dominance can occur during menopause if a woman is obese and has higher levels of estrogen due to estrone (E3) conversion into estradiol (E2).

Perimenopause

Perimenopause is the time surrounding the onset of menopause. It usually ranges from the ages of 38 to 55 depending upon when a woman stops menstruating or enters menopause. Menopause is defined as the cessation of a woman's menstrual cycles. In their late thirties, many women in the U.S. begin to experience changes in the premenstrual or *luteal phase* of their menstrual cycles. This time can be marked by an increase in emotional sensitivity, breast tenderness, abdominal bloating, and an increase in fatigue. Women's menstrual flows can be heavy due to the buildup of the uterine lining under the influence of estrogen with little to no progesterone to maintain it. This is a sign that the progesterone level is dropping and creating an imbalance in the estrogen to progesterone ratio. This imbalance also decreases progesterone's protective effects. This is the stage of perimenopause when women typically see their physicians for an increase in premenstrual symptoms and are frequently treated with oral contraceptives, antidepressants or both. This can exaggerate their symptoms, as oral contraceptives contain synthetic estrogen and progesterone, while antidepressants numb emotions. These synthetic treatments often increase the symptoms and risks caused by estrogen dominance. Women in this stage of perimenopause also need to understand how their lifestyle choices can influence their symptoms, the meaning of their symptoms and the therapeutic options available.

Additional symptoms of perimenopause

As a woman advances into her forties, her physical symptoms can increase if hormone imbalance is either ignored or exaggerated with the use of synthetic hormones. This can aggravate estrogen dominance. Some of these symptoms are:

- insomnia
- hot flashes
- night sweats
- depression
- anxiety
- hair thinning
- heavy menstrual flow
- bowel spasms, constipation and diarrhea (irritable bowel syndrome)
- dry skin
- joint pain
- joint stiffness
- muscle pain
- weight gain
- fatigue
- hair loss
- loss of libido
- urinary incontinence
- acid reflux
- hypertension
- headaches
- nausea
- food sensitivities
- allergies
- increased in fat production
- increase in blood sugar
- mild vertigo (dizziness)

Between ages 45 and 55, women begin to experience a decline in estrogen levels as the ovaries continue to wind down. As estrogen *decreases*, symptoms of hot flashes and night sweats can increase due to the withdrawal that estrogen receptors experience from reduced levels of estrogen. Additionally, in the U.S., where women eat more processed than whole foods, their bodies become depleted of energy. Both of these causes can lead to significant reductions in energy and vitality.

For most women, changes in diet that include more earth-based and animal-free foods in combination with natural progesterone prescribed by their physicians can moderately reduce their peri-menopausal symptoms. Often the addition of natural progesterone can cause an additional decrease in symptoms caused by declining estrogen levels due to its mildly estrogenic effects. If natural proges-terone does not improve these symptoms of estrogen withdrawal, a small dose of natural estrogen may be needed for symptom man-agement and balance.

Post menopausal symptoms and replacement of synthetic estrogen with natural estrogen

Traditional medicine defines a woman as post-menopausal if she has not menstruated for one year. Women who no longer men-struate and suffer from severe hot flashes and night sweats can be helped with a low dose of natural estrogen if natural progesterone alone does not relieve their symptoms. In most women, a small dose of natural estrogen will be adequate to decrease their meno-pausal symptoms and offer only minimal risk. It should always be balanced with natural progesterone to decrease the risks and symp-toms of estrogen dominance.

If a woman is on synthetic hormone replacement (HRT) and wants to switch to natural hormones, an effective regimen is to begin natural estrogen at doses equivalent to the synthetic estro-gen she is taking. Natural estrogen has a more gentle effect on the body than synthetic estrogen, so initially a slightly higher dose is sometimes needed as her body may have symptoms of withdrawal if equivalent doses of natural to synthetic hormones are taken. Once a woman has been on a prescribed dose of natural estrogen for a month or two and is asymptomatic, she can begin a gradual weaning of it under the guidance of her physician. The goal is to obtain hormone *balance*, and not replace hormones at menstrual levels, as balance carries less probability for estrogen dominance and its associated risks. Moreover, as estrogen levels decline with age, estrogen receptors in women's bodies are unable to process high levels of estrogen. The hormone receptor function decreases since hormones are biologically programmed to decline. Estrogen receptors incorporate estrogen into cells. If *menstrual* doses of estrogen are administered during perimenopause and especially menopause for *replacement*, their side effects and risks increase.

The strategy of gradual weaning of natural estrogen enables the estrogen receptor to get used to lower levels of estrogen over time, minimizing a woman's estrogen withdrawal symptoms. The goal is to use the least amount of estrogen required for symptom relief. Plant-based estrogens or phytoestrogens (*plant based estrogens*) such as organic soy and preferably fermented soy are also very effective for symptomatic relief from estrogen withdrawal. Pills and bars containing soy may not be as safe to take because soy in this form does not have as much of a protective effect and may actually stimulate the estrogen receptor. If a woman is unable to tolerate natural hormone therapy, phytoestrogens can also offer her relief and protection from overstimulation of the estrogen receptor, reducing the symptoms of estrogen dominance.

Progesterone and mood

As the progesterone level declines, so does the serotonin level in the brain and body. Serotonin is a chemical produced by the nervous system that regulates mood, sleep, appetite, learning and muscle contractions in large muscles and the gut. It contributes to feelings of well-being. When its levels decline, we may feel depressed, anxious, have difficulty staying asleep, and have bloating and irritability of the bowels. Progesterone increases the level of serotonin in the brain and nervous system. As progesterone declines, the level of serotonin decreases, resulting in the symptoms of mild depression and anxiety. In addition, estrogen *decreases* levels of serotonin in the brain. These can be replenished with natural progesterone. Many physicians treat depression caused by estrogen dominance during perimenopause with antidepressants rather than natural progesterone.

Synthetic progesterone

The traditional medical system prescribes synthetic progesterone or *Progestin*, as a form of hormone replacement therapy for menopause. Synthetic progesterone is manufactured in a laboratory and does not have the same chemical structure as natural progesterone (figure 2). Natural or bioidentical progesterone's chemical structure is identical to progesterone produced in a woman's body. Synthetic progesterone is not able to correct estrogen dominance. It is also dangerous for women to take. A large scale Women's Health Initiative study, conducted in the U.S. in 1998, was halted three years early in 2002 when it showed that the combination of synthetic estrogen and synthetic progesterone (progestin) increased a woman's risk of heart disease, breast cancer and strokes. Unfortunately, despite this evidence, prescribing practices for synthetic hormones in the U.S. have not changed and physicians continue to prescribe them for menopausal symptoms.

Natural hormone therapy

In my years of helping women transition through menopause, I have had the opportunity to observe which treatments are effective, and which offer minimal to no benefit. I have concluded that women feel better when their hormones are balanced. In addition, hormone balance lowers the incidence of menopausal symptoms and the risks of diseases caused by estrogen dominance.

Using a common sense approach to treatment and balance is usually the best way to navigate through menopause. If women can view their symptoms from the framework of estrogen dominance, they can minimize their intake of synthetic estrogen and supplement with natural progesterone as prescribed by their physicians in order to maintain balance and improve health.

As shown by The Women's Health Initiative study, *synthetic* progesterone (progestin) does not carry the safety we have been told that it does. Synthetic hormones have significantly different effects on the body than natural hormones. Even a small difference in molecular structure can cause a significant difference in efficacy, risk and side effects. Synthetic progesterone has a different molecular structure than natural progesterone (figure 2). Natural progesterone has a molecular structure that is identical to a woman's body and is much safer to take than synthetic progesterone. If it wasn't, our body would not produce it.

Numerous studies published in the medical literature over the past two decades have supported the beneficial effects of natural progesterone. The majority of these studies have been published in the European medical literature.

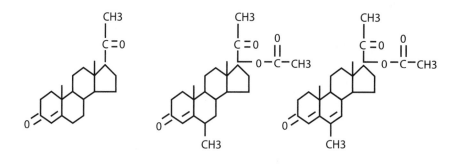

Natural progesterone   Progestin (synthetic)   Provera (synthetic)

Figure 2: Differences between the molecular structures
of natural and synthetic progesterone

Compounding pharmacy

A *compounding pharmacy* is a pharmacy where natural or bioidentical hormones are available with a prescription from a physician. *Bioidentical is identical to what your body produces* (figure 2). Natural progesterone is progesterone derived from wild yams or soybeans. A substance called diosgenin is extracted from them which is synthesized into a substance with the same molecular structure as progesterone produced by human ovaries and adrenal glands. Natural estrogen, progesterone and testosterone are all available from a compounding pharmacy.

Synthetic vs natural hormones

As synthetic hormones do not share the molecular structure of natural hormones they can be patented and sold by the pharmaceutical industry. Natural substances cannot be patented. Synthetic hormones are recognized and processed by the body differently than bioidentical hormones. This is what causes their side effects and risks. This creates toxicity in the body rather than balance. Since the liver is not equipped to process synthetic substances, it cannot adequately break down and eliminate them. Traces of them are stored in fatty tissues that can lead to health problems. Additionally, synthetic hormones have the effect of suppressing natural hormones produced by the ovaries.

Synthetic progesterone is termed *Progestin*. This should not be confused with *progesterone*. Unopposed synthetic estrogen (estrogen without progesterone), prescribed by the health care system is a contributing factor to the peri- and post-menopausal symptoms in the U.S. This is prescribed primarily in women who have had hysterectomies and are on synthetic hormone replacement therapy consisting of only synthetic estrogen.

A woman on five or more years of synthetic hormone replacement therapy has a 66% increased risk of breast cancer and a 22%

increased risk of death. Numerous studies performed since 1989 and published in traditional medical journals in the U.S. have consistently shown significant health risks for women who use synthetic hormones *for up to 10 years after their discontinuation*. The risk of breast, uterine and ovarian cancers, as well as, strokes and heart attacks increases and these risks must be considered before taking any synthetic hormone replacement therapy.

Natural progesterone

The hormone that women need most during the perimenopausal years is natural or bioidentical progesterone. Women continue to produce estrogen during this time, but as the progesterone level declines from the inconsistency of ovulation with age, symptoms of estrogen dominance become more frequent, particularly during the *luteal phase* of the menstrual cycle. It is critical to measure hormone blood levels periodically and regulate the dosage of natural progesterone based on a woman's clinical response in order to maintain estrogen and progesterone balance and ensure safe dosing. High doses of hormones can carry health risks. *Balance* is the goal of natural hormone therapy. *Balance* is achieved with the lowest doses of natural hormones that can lead to symptomatic improvement. Menstrual doses of hormones administered during perimenopause and menopause may carry potential danger of side effects and health risks. It is not natural for women going through menopause to take doses of hormones that result in menstrual levels of estrogen and progesterone.

For most women, the initial effects of natural progesterone can be felt as early as two days after starting it. A woman will find that her sleep cycle becomes more regular and she will frequently begin to experience deeper and a more restful night's sleep. She awakens less often and when she does, she is able to fall back to sleep again. With the sleep cycle restored, her stress hormones decline, and she feels more rested and vital.

Women often begin to feel more grounded and emotionally balanced within a few days of taking natural progesterone. After taking it for a few months, symptoms of estrogen dominance are significantly reduced. Women find that it is easier to lose weight once hormone balance is attained, as the thyroid works more efficiently when the hormones are balanced. Estrogen dominance can lead to mild suppression of thyroid function that decreases metabolism and increases weight. In addition, estrogen increases the accumulation of body fat by reducing the body's ability to break down fat and increasing the body's production of fat. Progesterone counterbalances the fat stimulating effects of estrogen.

Natural progesterone:

- acts as a mild diuretic decreasing water retention
- relaxes the intestines decreasing bloating and constipation
- improves the integrity of hair, skin and muscles
- regulates the sleep cycle
- reduces anxiety and depression
- decreases heavy menstrual flow
- regulates the insulin receptor increasing the efficiency of sugar metabolism
- clears foggy thinking
- improves memory
- relaxes blood vessels lowering blood pressure
- reduces fatigue
- promotes weight loss
- improves thyroid function

Dosing of progesterone

The dosing of progesterone should be regulated under the guidance of a physician who has experience in prescribing natural hormones with objective laboratory monitoring. Many brands of natural progesterone that are available over the counter and by mail order have very low doses of progesterone that may not provide adequate balance during perimenopause. Sometimes over-the-counter brands have not been compounded to bioidentical progesterone, preventing it from being therapeutically available to the body for balance.

The dosage of natural progesterone required for balance should be determined by your physician, based on your blood levels and clinical response. Most women experience feelings of well-being and significant reductions in symptoms caused by estrogen dominance. The usual prescribed dose of natural progesterone ranges from 12.5mg to 200mg per day. It is available in the form of a cream, gel, capsule or sublingual drops. Your physician can help determine the form that works best for you. If you are still cycling, natural hormones are cycled in conjunction with the menstrual cycle, with progesterone being administered during the *luteal phase*. If you are post-menopausal, the dosage regimen of progesterone can be administered for either six out seven days per week, or up to 26 out of 30 days per month. If either or both natural testosterone and estrogen are prescribed, they are usually administered in daily dosing regimens.

Women who are overweight have a higher concentration of estrogen in their bodies, as fat cells produce estrone (E1). Estrone can convert into estradiol (E2). Sometimes women who have excess body fat initially need higher doses of progesterone in order to achieve balance, and their levels should be closely monitored to make sure that they are not converting progesterone to estrogen.

Some symptoms of high levels of natural progesterone may include increased sedation, bloating, weight gain, headaches, fatigue and breast tenderness.

As women become familiar with the process involved in restoring hormone balance and notice improvement in their symptoms when their hormones are balanced, they will be able to tell if they need additional blood levels checked between testing intervals. They will feel symptoms of imbalance if their blood levels on natural hormones are too high or too low. They may experience symptoms of headaches, bloating and fatigue if their progesterone level is too high, or they may experience symptoms of estrogen dominance if their progesterone level is too low or estrogen level is too high. This would indicate the need for a dose adjustment.

My patients often inform me when they feel the need for a dose adjustment between established testing intervals. In the majority of cases, they are correct. If they feel balanced and stable on a regimen that indicates an ideal ratio of estrogen to progesterone, they should have their levels checked every three months. If they achieve levels of hormone balance that remain stable and they remain asymptomatic, the time interval between testing can be slightly prolonged.

Natural estrogen

Most women produce small amounts of estrogen throughout their lives. In most cases, estrogen levels are higher in women who are moderately obese compared to thinner women.

Estrogen *replacement* is rarely needed in peri- and post-menopausal women. The most common situation requiring estrogen *replacement* is in a woman who has had a complete hysterectomy (uterus and ovarian removal). It is a shock for the body to go through surgical menopause and hormone receptors often can go through moderate to severe hormone withdrawal. Women in these situations need natural estrogen *replacement,* if they experience severe hot flashes, night sweats and extreme insomnia. The replacement doses of estrogen can be gradually weaned over time. It is important to always combine natural estrogen replacement with natural progesterone and testosterone as the ovaries are no longer present to transition a woman gradually through perimenopause. An additional reason for using natural estrogen would be to replace prescribed synthetic estrogen as a safer alternative and then to gradually wean it as tolerated.

Women who suffer from severe hot flashes and night sweats are sometimes helped with low doses of natural estrogen. It is important to try not to *replace* the estrogen levels, given that there are long-standing potential risks of using high doses of estrogen taken during perimenopause and menopause. This must always be done under the guidance of a physician who monitors blood levels of estrogen to maintain safety.

Hormone imbalance and withdrawal can often cause adrenal stress that increases symptoms of exhaustion and fatigue. It can also lead to adrenal burnout where the adrenal glands are unable to mount an adequate level of hormones necessary for health and well-being. Both physicians and patients need to weigh the consequences of adrenal stress that accompanies severe menopausal symptoms caused by low estrogen levels against the risks of estrogen use.

Estriol cream

As mentioned earlier, estriol (E3) is a form of estrogen that is produced almost exclusively during pregnancy by the developing fetus. It crosses the placental barrier and enters the mother's body during pregnancy. It has been found to be safer than estradiol (E2), in women who are not pregnant, and it carries a much lower risk of uterine and breast cancer than estradiol. Estriol provides benefits to the vagina, cervix and vulva. When vaginal atrophy results from the absence of estrogen, it can lead to symptoms of pain, bleeding, cystitis and painful intercourse. Vaginal insertion of estriol in the form of a cream is helpful in restoring moisture and reducing the occurrence of urethral and bladder inflammation. Since it is not the primary estrogen present in the body affecting the breast and uterine tissue, it is safer than estradiol and effective for restoring the vaginal mucosal lining. It undergoes conversion to estradiol in only small amounts in a woman's body.

DHEA

DHEA is a vital adrenal hormone, which is a precursor of estrogen, progesterone and testosterone. Under conditions of chronic stress, and adrenal fatigue, DHEA levels can fall. A blood test can measure its levels and multiple levels measured during the day give the most accurate reading of DHEA. The morning level can provide adequate information to determine whether adrenal stress is present and whether DHEA supplementation is needed.

Short term supplementation to balance DHEA levels can be extremely helpful in decreasing fatigue and restoring vitality. DHEA is available as an over-the-counter supplement, but should only be used for short periods of time at low doses and under the guidance of a physician. It should be weaned once its levels rise and blood levels should be carefully monitored. When DHEA is taken without supervision, it can increase the risk of hormone sensitive cancers.

Any level of chronic stress can lead to adrenal fatigue. Once the stress is managed and passes, the adrenals can recover and DHEA levels are quickly restored. The body is extremely resilient when cared for with an understanding of how to support its process.

As we learn more about the positive effects of natural or bioidentical hormones and the protection they provide for midlife women, we will be able to safely take them for the menopausal transition in order to maintain balance and vitality. Until clinical research in the U.S. is funded to study their effects, many traditional physicians may continue to resist prescribing natural hormones to their patients. We must rely on common sense and the clinical experience of physicians who have prescribed these hormones for years in their patient populations. The data available from European studies offers scientific guidance for prescribing natural hormones safely. In addition, European studies have demonstrated the safety of natural hormones over a significant period of time. Given the highly estrogenic environment in the U.S. that differs from other countries research done here would need to be more specific and applicable to our population of women.

All hormone usage carries a level of risk. The field of natural hormone therapy is one that continues to evolve and grow. We must remain informed and stay open minded while using science as our guide for exploring the use and safety of natural hormones. Natural hormones have been shown to carry less risk than synthetic hormones. However, they should only be taken under the close guidance of physicians who follow scientific method and high standard-of-care and are skilled in prescribing and balancing them.

4

Food as Medicine

Let food be your medicine and medicine be your food.
~Hippocrates, 390 B.C.

Our cultural relationship with food has a profound influence on our personal relationship with it. In many parts of the world, sharing a meal is central to the physical and emotional nourishment of family and community. It is at the heart of the dinner table and the focus of social gatherings. It is a catalyst for connection. It is considered a form of art and a basis for health in most of the world. Food is grown and prepared with care when it is considered central to health and well-being. People living in cultures where food is valued are healthier and happier.

American's have a dysfunctional relationship with food. It is not considered integral to health. Food is not valued by our health care system. It is not seen as a form of art or nourishment. It is not central to our time together at the dinner table. We are the country that created "fast food." In addition, eating is a highly charged emotional issue for us. Our focus is on dieting, not nourishment, on weight loss, not health. Food is associated with feelings of failure and shame, and the relationship that many American women have with it is far from sacred. Physicians receive little or no training in nutrition. Hospital dieticians are not ecologically focused and follow health guidelines dictated by corporate health care and "agribusiness" which lack ecological and sustainable perspectives. They do not educate their patients to consider food as central to promoting health. Instead, they focus on its calorie content. This activates fear of its consumption. They give emphasis to quantity over quality. Our relationship with food needs to be reframed and healed in order for our society to become healthy. We need to realize that food and health are intrinsically related.

Europe is better at this relationship than we are. Food is central to their culture. Europeans began the "slow food" movement. They drew this from their experience of generations that considered food as the cause of health and vitality. This promoted a lifestyle that supported health and well-being. Being an integral part of their culture, it does not take much effort for Europeans to have a positive and healing relationship with food. It is the same for people from other parts of the world. Other cultures understand the importance of a healthy diet and lifestyle for health and well-being.

In the U.S., the food consumed is largely synthetic and processed. It takes effort and added expense to eat whole foods that are unprocessed and organically grown. Preparing and eating meals is considered a chore. Preparing meals takes time. People seek to maximize their time on more "productive" pursuits than cooking. Our relationship with food lacks heart and understanding. It lacks consciousness. We need awareness to understand that when we eat unnatural and processed foods, we are not fulfilled or satisfied. Because in our country, a positive association between food and health is lacking, our relationship with food has become dysfunctional. This kind of relationship does not nourish or sustain us at any level. We consume larger volumes of food than in order to compensate for our lack of satiety while eating processed and synthetic foods with "empty calories." These calories are derived from sugars and starches that are heavily processed and added to enhance flavor. People become addicted to these high sugar containing foods which affect their physiology and mood. This results in patterns of overconsumption of unhealthy foods which cause obesity and health problems, currently epidemic in our country. In our country, going on a diet is viewed as a solution to this problem.

The diet industry is a multibillion dollar industry that has a 97% failure rate. It is called the "Diet and Weight Loss" industry. It is based on controlling the *volume* of food and does not emphasize the importance of the *quality* of food for nourishment and health. It does not attempt to heal our unhealthy relationship with food; rather, it polarizes it. Food becomes our enemy that we work hard to avoid.

Midlife is a time when this relationship can become a central focus. During midlife, women's bodies begin to change. As they lose muscle tone some of which is replaced with fat, their caloric needs decrease. In addition, they may become less active due to fatigue and perimenopausal symptoms. When their hormones become imbalanced creating a state of chronic stress, women often lose their vitality and vigor. As they age they often feel lethargic and chronically fatigued. Due to fatigue, they have less control over their appetites. They eat in order to obtain extra energy and they also eat to compensate for their emotional hunger. It is the only way they know how to comfort themselves, as society does not offer them a healthy framework for emotional support. Physical food is not emotionally sustaining and they often eat rich and sweet comfort foods to medicate their feelings. When they eat this way, they do not provide their bodies with *needed* nourishment. They eat what they *want*. This leaves their bodies malnourished and craving for needed nutrients. Their bodies stay hungry for these nutrients they rarely get due to their lack of awareness. They confuse the body's appetite for nourishment with their appetite for emotional comfort. Over time, this becomes a pattern of their relationship with food.

This problem is epidemic amongst midlife women. Physicians do not address these issues that are central to Women's Health and many women suffer in silence. They are unable to access the self-care needed for self-control when they feel stressed and they have nowhere safe to go for a healthy approach to nutritional advice and weight loss. They find their way to many narrowly focused diet and weight loss programs, where they may feel the pressure to succeed at losing weight, and shame when they don't. Hospital dieticians offer food protocols that are difficult to follow, and women are afraid to admit their struggles to them due to the shame they feel. Unless we explore this dilemma to uncover and understand it, we will be unable to find lasting solutions to our health. This topic is of great importance for midlife women. My hope is to shed light on some of these issues in order to release the distortions that are currently present in our relationship with food, and restore it to one that is healthy and whole. In order to achieve this goal, we need to begin by understanding how food affects our bodies and our health; which foods promote health, and how our emotional well-being influences our relationship with food.

The effect of food on the midlife body

In order for us to support our bodies, it is important to understand our changing body's needs. This understanding can provide the awareness required to make choices that promote health and vitality. Midlife marks a time when the switch to natural, organic and earth-based foods becomes critical for restoring health. Because cells are more vulnerable under the influence of changing hormones, the chemical make-up, energy and vitality of the foods consumed has a greater impact on them. Similarly, if unhealthy foods are eaten, they negatively influence the body's cell structure and increase vulnerability to illness. The body is always searching to heal and repair cell damage. Due to the increased biological sensitivity present in the midlife body, when whole foods are added to the diet, it is able to repair cell damage resulting from unhealthy foods consumed in the past.

The sensitive midlife body

The body becomes more sensitive in midlife under the influence of hormonal changes. Cell receptor sensitivity increases and women become vulnerable to the symptoms caused by a variety of foods such as gluten, dairy, sugar and alcohol. Many women are unable to tolerate these foods in midlife. In my medical practice, I advise women who complain of foggy thinking and lack of energy to try a diet free of gluten, alcohol and processed foods for three months, while also reducing their intake of dairy and processed sugar. In seventy five percent of them, moderately reducing or eliminating these foods alone restores their clarity and vitality. A large majority of women also lose significant amounts of weight. Their hot flashes and night sweats improve, and their skin becomes supple and vibrant. As they introduce root vegetables, greens, brown rice and quinoa into their diets, they begin to experience an increase in energy and resilience. Most of these foods have been shown in clinical studies to have cholesterol lowering effects, as well as reductions in the risk of heart disease and diabetes. Women's cholesterol levels can drop as much as 100 points without medications when these dietary changes are made.

Dietary influences on estrogen dominance

Estrogen dominance is aggravated by the pesticide-laden processed foods we eat, as pesticide residues on plants have estrogenic effects on the body. These are the xenoestrogens mentioned in chapter 3. Meat and dairy is laden with hormone residues that accumulate in the body and widen the level of estrogen and progesterone imbalance. The epidemic use of synthetic hormones in agribusiness, as well as, their rising concentrations in the groundwater from animal runoff and in the urine of women taking synthetic hormones and oral contraceptives, creates an unhealthy environment that puts all at risk for estrogen dominance. It makes us vulnerable to breast and uterine cancers, fibroids, endometriosis, hypothyroidism and a myriad of symptoms including insulin resistance, hypertension, weight gain and heart disease. Estrogen dominance opposes the thyroid and decreases metabolic drive, creating a losing battle for women who are attempting to lose weight with calorie control and exercise alone. Physicians rarely, if ever, mention these factors that contribute to menopausal symptoms. The addition of synthetic hormone replacement for the management of perimenopausal symptoms in midlife often aggravates a woman's risk of estrogen dominance and its associated risks.

Heart disease in women

Heart disease is the leading cause of death among American women. Despite growing advances in technological medicine, a quarter of all deaths before the age of sixty-five are from heart attacks. Inflammatory foods are the leading cause of coronary artery disease. When we eat foods high in sugar or simple carbohydrates (which break down to sugar in the body), the arteries become inflamed. Most of these foods are rich in saturated fat and partially hydrogenated oils that accelerate the formation of coronary plaque. This also increases blood cholesterol levels for which cholesterol lowering medications are prescribed. High cholesterol is NOT a risk factor in over half of our heart attacks. Despite this fact, cholesterol-lowering medications are some of the most frequently prescribed medications in midlife. In the health care system, nutrition and lifestyle are not emphasized as treatments of heart disease and its related risk factors, but as *accessory* components in disease prevention and health promotion. Physicians who do not inform their patients about the importance of lifestyle modification for the prevention and treatment of illness cannot make an impact on preventing future occurrence of heart disease, except with prescription drugs. Moreover, insurance companies do not cover office visits for preventative medicine practiced by physicians. Physicians are not compensated for time spent educating their patients. Patients are left to educate themselves about these issues. It is vitally important that patients educate and empower themselves with the information available on the significant influences that lifestyle can have on health.

It was believed for decades that the fall in estrogen levels after menopause was the cause for an increased incidence of heart attacks. Premenopausal women have fewer heart attack deaths than post-menopausal women. The more likely hormonal culprit is not the lack of estrogen, but the lack of *progesterone*. This has been shown in numerous studies in Europe. My clinical observation is that women become more sensitive to cellular wear and tear from stress hormones due to falling progesterone levels and estrogen dominance. Their bodies manifest illness with greater intensity after menopause if inflammatory foods are a large part of their diets. When women are stressed, adrenalin and cortisol levels, the main stress hormones, increase in the bloodstream. Often, these cause small tears in the coronary arteries that become foci for plaque formation. Stress hormones also cause coronary artery spasm. Under their influence, a 20 to 30% occlusion in an artery can clamp down to a 100% closure causing a heart attack or coronary event. Natural progesterone relaxes the coronary arteries and reduces arterial spasm that can lead to heart attacks. It also increases the beneficial cholesterol, HDL, which when present at high levels, is able to clear harmful cholesterol from the body.

Multiple studies have shown that *synthetic* estrogen and *synthetic* progesterone (progestin) increase the risk of spasm in the coronary arteries. Many physicians do not differentiate between synthetic and natural progesterone and do not prescribe the latter, leading to a perpetuation of estrogen dominance from synthetic hormone replacement, and its associated symptoms and risks.

With the burgeoning amount of information available about food and nutrition, women become confused about what diets to follow, what supplements to take and how to weave lifestyle changes that consist of whole foods into their pantries, refrigerators and bodies. For some, this is the first time in their lives when they learn about healthy eating. Many of my midlife patients have spent most of their lives eating prepared and processed foods purchased from the freezer sections in grocery stores and heated in microwave ovens. Eating in this manner aggravates estrogen dominance and its associated menopausal symptoms. Many women lack the experience of cooking whole foods and become used to eating prepared and processed foods. They must learn the association between food and health, the importance of true nourishment and the healing power of whole foods.

Easy food rules

The educational framework that is most successful in my medical practice is a simple one—eating needs to be easy, simple and fun. The following points can be helpful in creating a nutritional plan that is easy, fast and simple and can provide maximal benefits to promote health:

1. Half of your plate should have color, the color of organic vegetables—green, orange, red, purple or yellow.

2. A quarter of your plate should contain an organic protein rich food, preferably fish (not farmed), hormone and antibiotic free free-range chicken, beans, lentils or tofu, with minimal to no red meat.

3. A quarter of your plate should have an organic complex carbohydrate such as brown rice, quinoa, and wild rice or pasta. Any white colored processed foods made with white flour or white rice should be minimized (figure 3).

4. Eat nuts and seeds between meals and eat small amounts of dark chocolate if sugar cravings are intense.

5. Drink no more than one cup of organic coffee per day, plenty of water (6 to 8 glasses of filtered water, preferably not from a plastic bottle) and green tea.

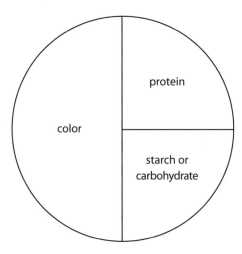

Figure 3: The optimum plate

6. Eat a handful of organic berries. Blueberries and strawberries are the most nutrient dense.

7. The darker and deeper the color of food is in its natural form, the richer it is in antioxidants.

8. Eat plenty of organic root vegetables. Always remember to eat organically grown vegetables because root vegetables are scavengers that keep the soil clean by absorbing pesticides from it more than other vegetables.

9. Eat moderate amounts of *organic* soy. A recent study from China performed with 5000 women ages 25–75 with estrogen positive and negative breast cancers divided the women into two groups. One group ate 5g or less of soy per day, and the other group ate 12g or more of soy per day. The results showed a 30% reduction in mortality in the group that ate 12g or more of soy per day as part of their diets. Soy is a *phytoestrogen* or a plant-based estrogen. Phytoestrogens are effective in reducing menopausal symptoms and decreasing a woman's risk of breast cancer. However, it is necessary to consume only *organic* soy, as non-organic

soy is heavily sprayed with pesticides and a large percentage of it is genetically modified.

The optimum plate

Diets often fail because they are complicated and have too many rules to follow. It is important to keep our relationship with food simple. Living in harmony with nature and consuming mostly earth-based foods is a way to accomplish this.

My patients have greatly benefited from simplifying their diets with an understanding of how to divide their plates. An easy way to make sure you are getting a balanced diet, as mentioned before is to divide your plate into three sections. First divide it in half and then divide one half into two quarters. Half of the plate should contain foods with color such as dark vegetables; a quarter should contain protein and a quarter should contain a complex carbohydrate (figure 3). If two meals a day are eaten according to this formula, women will get 80% more nutrition than they are currently receiving from their diets.

Good rules of thumb:

• Dark fruits and vegetables have plenty of cancer fighting properties. Eat a variety of them daily.

• Dark leafy greens such as kale, collards, Swiss chard, romaine lettuce and spinach are nutrient rich. Kale is the most nutrient dense green you can eat, packing beta carotene, vitamin K and C, lutein, calcium and sulforaphane (a chemical with potent anti-cancer properties).

• Minimize intake of acidic foods such as dairy and red meat. All animal protein creates an acidic environment in the body. In order to neutralize the acidity, the body draws calcium from the bones, increasing bone loss. Over time, this causes a reduction in bone density which can lead to osteopenia and osteoporosis, diseases epidemic in the U.S.

• Refined sugar is toxic to the body.

• Obtain information on nutrition and health from reputable nutrition books, not television advertisements for processed foods.

• Eat foods from the produce shelf in the far end of the grocery store, not from a box. Boxed foods are processed. Most foods located in the middle aisles of a grocery store are processed.

• Eat as much local organic produce as possible. It has less of a chance of being nutrient poor. Produce shipped from long distances loses its nutritional content over time spent in transport. In addition, you will be supporting local organic farmers and sustainable farming practices.

• Minimize salt intake.

• Replace butter and margarine for cooking with monounsaturated and polyunsaturated oils such as olive oil and canola or safflower oil.

• Eat whole grains and a variety of nuts and seeds.

• Minimize the intake of gluten rich foods such as wheat and white bread, cookies and crackers and white flour based pasta.

• Replace foods containing processed flour with sprouted substitutes.

• Keep portion sizes small and eat until you are no longer hungry. This will require you to remain conscious while eating.

• Avoid foods that are high in pesticide residues. The best way to avoid eating them is to eat organic fruits and vegetables. The following fruits and vegetables called "the dirty dozen," are classified as containing the highest concentrations of pesticide residues:

1. Celery
2. Peaches
3. Strawberries
4. Apples
5. Blueberries
6. Nectarines
7. Bell peppers
8. Spinach
9. Kale
10. Cherries
11. Potatoes
12. Grapes

Insulin resistance

The body produces a hormone called insulin in response to a sugar load from a meal. The main sources of sugars consumed in the U.S. are refined sugars and simple carbohydrates in the form of bread, pasta, snacks and desserts. Carbohydrates break down to sugar in the body. Insulin is required to mobilize sugar into cells where it can be used for energy. If a person eats a large amount of sugar or carbohydrate containing foods, the body does not need to use up its fat stores for energy, especially when regular exercise is not part of one's lifestyle.

When sugar or glucose enters the body, it signals the pancreas to produce a hormone called insulin. Insulin levels rise with increases in blood sugar. Insulin's role is to keep the blood sugar in the body within a narrow range. Blood sugar levels above this range can be toxic to cells. Insulin converts excess blood sugar into a sugar storage compound called glycogen and stores it in the liver and muscles. If the blood sugar is too high, it is converted to fat and stored in fatty tissue.

In metabolic syndrome, as large quantities of sugar or glucose enter the body, the body secretes large amounts of insulin due to high sugar intake and lack of exercise. Over time, this causes the common condition called insulin resistance. Glucose or sugar levels rise in the blood, signaling the production of more insulin. This creates a vicious cycle resulting in high levels of *both* glucose and insulin, which increases cholesterol, blood pressure, belly fat and arterial plaque. It is believed that 60% of heart disease in women is caused by insulin resistance.

High levels of insulin and sugar also increases the production of androgens or male hormones in the female body, thereby increasing the conversion of these androgens to estrogen, which aggravates estrogen dominance, leading to *Polycystic Ovarian Syndrome (PCOS)*. Women with PCOS have difficult and irregular menstrual cycles and a higher incidence of obesity, hypertension and insulin resistance. They also have a higher incidence of infertility.

Insulin resistance is a precursor to:

- diabetes
- heart disease
- high cholesterol
- abdominal obesity
- estrogen dominance
- fatigue
- hypothyroidism
- water retention
- hypertension
- irregular menses
- polycystic ovarian syndrome

To counteract this cycle and decrease insulin resistance, a healthy diet consisting of ample vegetables, fiber, protein and complex carbohydrates is necessary. We need to eat more whole foods and less processed carbohydrates and sugars, in order to maintain our health and prevent the development of insulin resistance.

Gluten sensitivity

Gluten sensitivity has become a rising health condition and concern in midlife in the U.S. Gluten is a protein contained in flour that creates the elasticity present in dough. Decades ago, our wheat grinding process preserved the oils in wheat. Since wheat was coarse, when eaten, gluten was not released in high concentrations into the blood stream. In contrast, today's wheat processing methods pulverize the wheat berry destroying its integrity and releases high concentrations of gluten into flour. When we eat foods containing white flour processed in this manner, the gluten contained in it is easily released into our bloodstream. Bread, processed crackers, cookies and baked goods contain high concentrations of gluten. Oats, barley and rye may contain small amounts of gluten. If you are sensitive to gluten, you can tell by the way you feel after eating a meal that is high in gluten. If you feel mental fog or drowsiness, you are most likely gluten sensitive.

Gluten can cause irritable bowel symptoms such as intestinal spasms and irregular bowel movements, in addition to abdominal bloating. Gluten sensitivity has been also been associated with symptoms of depression and anxiety, as well as, neurological symptoms such as numbness and tingling. It can cause skin rashes and weight gain. Some cases of mental illness have shown profound improvement when gluten has been eliminated from the diet.

There is a large amount of surface area present in the small intestine due to the folds that form its inner lining called "villi." Their function is to help us absorb nutrients from food. When a person is gluten sensitive, villi become flattened due to inflammation and breakdown. This causes a loss of the intestinal surface area, which decreases the absorption of nutrients, particularly iron and vitamin D.

Blood levels of iron and vitamin D can be measured by laboratory testing. If they are both low, despite the consumption of a balanced diet, it often indicates a degree of gluten intolerance. When gluten is eliminated from the diet of gluten sensitive individuals, the villi grow back within several months to a year and the surface area of the intestines is restored. This leads to a dramatic improvement in the symptoms of gluten intolerance. If gluten is reintroduced into the diet after eliminating it for a few months, exaggerated symptoms of mental fog and fatigue, bloating, weight gain and sometimes rashes may occur. In my medical practice, patients can quickly tell if they are gluten sensitive after eliminating gluten from their diets. They begin to think more clearly, lose weight and feel more energized.

The most conclusive test to determine gluten sensitivity is a small intestinal biopsy. Since this is costly and invasive, it is not recommended unless one's symptoms are severe. Discontinuing gluten for a period of one to two months and then reintroducing it with resulting symptom recurrence is a reliable test for gluten sensitivity or intolerance.

Celiac disease is a condition where gluten is considered a foreign substance by the body. With this disease, the body exhibits an inflammatory response upon ingestion of gluten. This can present with symptoms of severe rashes, diarrhea, irritable bowel symptoms, depression, anxiety, chronic fatigue and malabsorption and sometimes as mild symptoms of mental illness. A blood test can demonstrate if a person has celiac disease, although it may not be 100% definitive.

Prostaglandins

Prostaglandins are hormone-like substances that are derived from fats such as Omega-3 and Omega-6. Good fats create prostaglandins that are good for the body. These are called *series 1-prostaglandins*. They reduce the stickiness of blood and control blood cholesterol, improve immune function, maintain water balance, and reduce inflammation. Series 1-prostaglandins are derived through Omega-3 from fish, nuts and seeds. The highest concentrations of

Omega-3 can be found in mackerel and cold water fish like trout and salmon. All cold water fish are high in Omega-3.

Pro-inflammatory prostaglandins which synthesize *series 2-pros-taglandins* are found in animal fats, particularly red meat, dairy, corn oil, high-fructose corn syrup, or any kind of processed corn products, hydrogenated or trans-fats such as margarine and shortening and lard. These are directly linked to coronary plaque, as well as, many arthritic conditions. They are associated with inflammation and coronary thrombosis (*blood clots in the coronary arteries*). These are the prostaglandins that cause premenstrual syndrome (PMS) and uterine cramps. An effective way to heal the symptoms of menstrual cramping and PMS is to increase the intake of anti-inflammatory foods such as fresh vegetables and fruits, flax oil, nuts, seeds, legumes, whole grains, and extra virgin olive oil and Omega-3 and reduce the intake of animal and synthetically hydrogenated fats. High fructose corn syrup is highly inflammatory to cells and should be eliminated from the diet. Flax oil, fish, vegetables, nuts, seeds, organic eggs, whole grains and legumes should be increased. These modifications in food choices alone can significantly improve PMS and menstrual cramps as well as the common perimenopausal symptoms experienced by so many women in the U.S.

Supplements for the midlife woman

Some basic supplements to consider in the perimenopausal years are:

1. A multivitamin: A food-based multivitamin available at the health food store can deliver essential trace minerals and is easy to digest. It is important for it not to contain additives or chemical preservatives. It should be taken on a daily basis.

2. Vitamin D is a necessary vitamin shown in clinical studies to decrease the recurrence of breast cancer. It increases a woman's core

strength, builds bone density, and improves exercise tolerance. It is necessary to check blood levels if supplementing with this vitamin, as it is fat soluble and can become toxic if too much is taken and exceeds safe blood levels. In the Pacific Northwest and the Midwest, women have a need for greater doses of vitamin D in the winter months due to the prolonged lack of sun, since vitamin D is produced in the skin during sun exposure. The best food sources of vitamin D are herring, mackerel, salmon, oysters and eggs. The best vitamin D supplement is cholecalciferol or vitamin D3 of animal origin. Some physicians prescribe vitamin D in doses as high as 50,000 IU (international units) per month as a single dose. It is better to divide it into smaller daily doses taken over time and to monitor blood levels. The usual daily dose of vitamin D should be around 1000 to 2000 IUs per day.

In people who suffer from colitis or bowel disease, the risk of vitamin D deficiency is high due to malabsorption from intestinal inflammation. It is important to supplement with adequate doses of vitamin D3 to maintain a blood levels around 50 to 60. In women who are at risk for breast cancer or who have had breast cancer, maintaining this level is especially important in order to maintain health.

3. Vitamin E: Most food-based multivitamins contain an adequate daily supply of vitamin E (400 IUs per day). If one suffers from symptoms of breast tenderness and hot flashes, the addition of a vitamin E supplement can help ease these symptoms.

4. Omega-3 fish oil: Omega-3 is one of the most important supplements one can take. It is actually a supplement that everyone should take from cradle to grave. Our bodies do not produce DHA (docosahexaenoic acid), the active component of Omega-3, so we are dependent on food sources to obtain it. The richest food source for DHA is cold water fish. Our ancestors consumed a 1:1 ratio of Omega-3 to Omega-6 fatty acids. Omega-6 fatty acids are present in vegetable oils in addition to red meat and processed foods that compete with Omega-3 for space in the brain. Today Americans

consume an approximate ratio of 1:25 of Omega-3 to Omega-6, due to their heavy consumption of processed foods (made with Omega-6 rich fats and oils), and their low consumption of fish such as salmon, sardines that is rich in Omega-3. Krill is also high in Omega-3. Omega-3 has been shown to reduce the symptoms of PMS, particularly menstrual cramps and mild depression. Mood, emotions and mental concentration are adversely affected by low levels of Omega-3 in the diet. Omega-3 fats maintain the suppleness of the membranes surrounding the brain. They also increase the levels of dopamine and serotonin, two neurotransmitters when low are linked with depression, anxiety and addictive behavior. High levels of DHA present in fish oil supplements are critical to the promotion of health, and healthy brain function and development, in addition to the prevention of heart disease. DHA can also decrease joint inflammation, muscle pain and decrease the incidence of muscle and ligament injury. It has been shown to decrease total cholesterol, increase the level of HDL, and decrease the incidence of kidney disease, as well as symptoms of depression and anxiety.

An effective Omega-3 supplement should be pharmaceutically graded and micro distilled in order to remove potential traces of mercury, and should contain at least 300 mg of DHA per 1000 mg of Omega-3. I recommend taking 2000 mg of Omega-3, containing 600 mg of total DHA for daily maintenance. This has a blood-thinning effect, so it is important to talk with your physician about its safety while taking blood thinners, or if bleeding tendencies are present. Wild caught salmon has approximately 1000 mg of Omega-3 per 3 oz. serving. Farmed salmon does not contain high concentrations of Omega-3 and in addition, is high in pesticide residues as the salmon feed contains pesticides. Atlantic salmon has higher concentrations of mercury than Pacific, Norwegian or Alaskan salmon. Flax oil does not deliver DHA, although it has anti-inflammatory properties. Rather than DHA, it contains ALA (alpha linoleic acid), which does not have the same protective effects as DHA.

5. Magnesium is a beneficial supplement for women who suffer from leg cramps during perimenopause and menopause. Estrogen dominance can cause magnesium depletion resulting in these symptoms. Estrogen dominance increases the influx of water into the cells and causes the loss of potassium and magnesium from cells. This can lead to fatigue and muscle cramps. Moreover, the influx of water into cells can cause water weight gain, hypertension, and headaches. When natural progesterone is used in therapeutic doses, these symptoms dissipate and the addition of magnesium can ease the cramps and relax the muscles. It is not wise to add potassium to the supplement regimen unless the measured blood potassium is low and it is prescribed and monitored with blood levels. Too high or too low blood levels of potassium can result in fatal heart arrhythmias.

6. Calcium is used to build bones and to promote heart health. It is necessary for healthy cell membranes and muscle function. It is best to consume calcium from food sources rather than as a vitamin supplement. Calcium supplements have been linked with an increase in the formation of calcifications in the coronary arteries and breasts. The form of supplemental calcium best absorbed is calcium citrate combined with magnesium and boron. If you have osteopenia (moderate loss of bone density) or osteoporosis (significant loss of bone density), it is important to consult with your physician before starting a calcium supplement.

Caffeine, alcohol and acidifying foods such as meat and dairy, in addition to causing estrogen dominance causes the reduction of calcium in bones. The best sources of calcium are almonds, brewer's yeast, parsley, corn, artichokes, cooked dried beans, dark leafy greens and broccoli. Problems arising from excess calcium such as kidney stones can occur while taking excessive doses of calcium and vitamin D (if there is a predisposition to stone formation).

7. Vitamin C: Vitamin C strengthens the immune system and fights infections. It is a potent antioxidant that can protect the body

from cancer. The best food sources of vitamin C are peppers, broccoli, kiwi fruit, cabbage, watercress, strawberries, lemons, oranges and citrus fruits in general. Cigarette smoking, alcohol, fried foods and stress, rob the body of vitamin C. A 1000 to 2000mg Vitamin C supplement is recommended as a daily antioxidant.

Dietary influences of yin and yang balance

It is important to know that all foods contain energy. Traditional medicine divides food into categories such as fats, proteins and carbohydrates. It does not take into account the intrinsic energy that different foods contain and how this energy affects our bodies. If we acknowledged the importance of this in our culture, we would stop eating processed foods and only eat whole foods.

In Eastern traditions, the prevailing perspective is that the forces of Yin and Yang effect and shape everything in the world. Yin energy has cool, damp and dark qualities. It is the dark portion of the Yin and Yang symbol. Yang is warm, dry and light. It is the white part of the Yin and Yang symbol. The night is Yin; the day is Yang; winter is Yin; and summer is Yang. Cool is Yin; heat is Yang. Yin is the coolant for the Yang engine of the body.

All foods contain these energetic qualities. Yin and Yang energies need to be balanced in the body in order for us to be healthy and feel well. During perimenopause, Yin energy begins to recede resulting in the prominence of Yang energy. When Yin energy recedes, we experience the more common symptoms of perimenopause and menopause such as:

- hot flashes
- anxiety
- acid reflux
- dry hair
- night sweats
- hypertension
- dry skin
- skin rashes

Yin deficiency also causes fatigue that can to lead to sugar cravings. The body attempts to compensate for its lack of energy by making us crave sources of quick energy such as sugar and carbohydrate containing foods. Yin deficiency and Yang excess is common in the U.S. because the processed American diet is high in Yang energy. Processed foods, alcohol and meat are high in Yang energy, hence they tend to be warming, exaggerating the Yin and Yang imbalance and aggravating menopausal symptoms.

If we consider which foods contain high amounts of Yin or Yang energies, we can choose foods according to the nature of our symptoms. If we suffer from symptoms of high Yang energy such as hot flashes or night sweats, we can decrease these symptoms by increasing our intake of Yin foods. If we feel slow, sluggish and stagnant, we can eat more warming foods like spices, chicken, eggs and kale. It is recommended to eat more Yin (cooling) foods during midday and more Yang (warming) foods in the morning and evening. This is because the morning and evening are cooler and midday is warmer. Eating in this manner results in balancing the body's energy. More Yin foods should be eaten during the hot season and more Yang foods during the cool season. This is a helpful way to balance the body's energy.

Most perimenopausal women in midlife, suffer from Yin deficiency. The foods they eat should be higher in Yin energy to compensate for its loss. A practitioner trained in Traditional Chinese Medicine should be consulted to learn more about this discipline as a guide for designing a nutritional program to help with perimenopausal and menopausal symptoms.

Neutral foods are not high in either Yin or Yang energies. They are balanced and hence termed neutral.

Many women have strong reactions to alcohol and dairy during midlife. Their perimenopausal symptoms improve significantly when they minimize their intake of these foods. There is an overwhelming amount of evidence to suggest that an earth-based

YIN FOODS: calming, nourishing, cooling
Cucumber, daikon radish, eggplant, dandelion greens, romaine
lettuce, endive, spinach, millet, celery, cauliflower, bok choy,
apples, apricots, asparagus, carrots, Chinese cabbage, zucchini,
turnips, rutabaga, squash, watercress, cantaloupe, green tea,
seaweed

YANG FOODS: stimulating, energetic, warming
Meat, lamb, beef, chicken, cheese, salt, bell peppers, shrimp,
mustard greens, onions, scallions, chives, garlic, egg yolks,
leeks and kale

NEUTRAL FOODS:
Beets, brown rice, buckwheat, chard, corn, fish, lettuce, peas,
string beans, sweet potatoes, taro root, turkey and yams

vegetarian diet is the best diet for preventing cancer and heart
disease. It is also high in Yin energy. As we choose our foods with
consciousness and with a basic understanding of how to keep our
energy balanced, we can promote health and vitality and prevent
most illnesses caused by unhealthy lifestyles.

Exercise
There is no substitute for regular aerobic exercise. It is a necessary
part of self-care. My recommendation is to do 30 minutes of aerobic exercise at least five to six times per week, even if it is divided
to accommodate a busy schedule. It is valuable to keep the exercise
routine variable and interesting in order to prevent boredom. It is
one of the best therapies for stress and it can help in weight loss,
cholesterol reduction and for an improvement in cardiac capacity.

Special food considerations for Women's Health:

Foods that heal Premenstrual Syndrome (PMS)

An estimated 97% of American women have PMS at some time in their lives. Dietary changes can have a significant effect on these symptoms. PMS is often triggered by an imbalance in hormones that cause estrogen dominance. Restoration of hormone balance is influenced by the types of food we eat in addition to natural hormone therapy. Foods high in animal or saturated fat are converted into reproductive hormones in the body. These can create an imbalance in the estrogen to progesterone ratio.

Some simple food facts can help us make healthier food choices to support our bodies during perimenopause:

- Cholesterol is a precursor to reproductive hormones. It is found in animal fats and can increase hormone levels leading to imbalance.

- Many symptoms of PMS are similar to symptoms of estrogen dominance.

- The liver needs B complex to break down excess estrogen. If the diet is lacking B vitamins (green vegetables), excess estrogen accumulates in the body.

- If one does not eat enough fiber, an increased amount of estrogen is absorbed by the intestines, as the lack of fiber slows down the transit time of food in the intestines. In other words, estrogen stays in the intestines for a longer time and higher concentrations of it are absorbed into the bloodstream, raising its levels in the blood.

- Xenoestrogens from non-organic or pesticide-sprayed foods can accumulate in the body.

- A diet of non-organic meat and dairy high in synthetic hormones will increase the body's estrogen content.

- A diet high in sugar, and low in whole foods, results in elevations of estrogen, insulin and blood sugar levels creating mood disturbances and symptoms of estrogen dominance. This can lead to PCOS, metabolic syndrome, diabetes, elevated cholesterol, inflammatory conditions, weight gain and feelings of sluggishness.

The *luteal phase* of the menstrual cycle is when sugar cravings are most prominent. This is due, in part, to Yin deficiency during this part of the cycle, in addition to estrogen dominance. A woman under chronic stress, who consumes a diet high in synthetic estrogens, will experience an exaggeration of PMS symptoms such as pelvic cramps, weight gain, fluid retention, breast tenderness, depression and anxiety.

Progesterone is a hormone with Yin properties. It is responsible for women's menstrual cycles and it is produced cyclically every month in menstruating women. Adequate levels of progesterone can help women feel grounded. Women feel "ungrounded" when its levels fall. Estrogen has Yang properties. It is produced steadily and not cyclically in women's bodies, and hot flashes and night sweats are common Yang symptoms that result from a drop in its levels during perimenopause.

Foods for menstrual symptoms

Cramps, low back pain, headaches, heavy menstrual flow and fatigue are common symptoms during menses in American women. Many of these symptoms are related to their diets that stimulate the production of series 2-prostaglandins. Red meat and dairy stimulate the production of series 2-prostaglandins, as they contain arachadonic acid, which gets converted into series 2-prostaglandin. Red meat has the highest levels of arachadonic acid followed by lamb, pork, and then chicken and turkey. It is wise to eat more vegetarian foods especially during the *luteal phase* of the menstrual cycle. A diet high in B vitamins and fiber decreases the incidence of estrogen dominance.

If your periods are heavy, you are most likely estrogen dominant. A small amount of natural progesterone under the guidance of a physician in combination with an organic diet is often helpful.

Foods for perimenopause and menopause

Women in Asian countries who eat a diet high in vegetables and soy with an abundance of Yin foods have fewer symptoms during the peri- and post-menopausal years. One can create Yin energy stores by eating a diet high in Yin foods during the ages of twenty to forty. These are called the "Yin years," when Yin energy is utilized for creative pursuits such as career building, having babies and creating families. Most of us in the U.S. eat quick energy foods (such as processed foods), high in Yang energy during these years and do not form the Yin energy stores that can support our bodies during midlife. It is likened to a Yin savings account that we can use during perimenopause when our Yin energy is receding. If we do not have Yin stores in our savings account, we are more likely to experience the symptoms of Yin deficiency.

Phytoestrogens

Phytoestrogens are plant based estrogens. Their molecular formula is similar to estrogen and they have a mild estrogenic effect on the body. They also have the effect of decreasing the stimulation of estrogen receptors on cells. Contrary to the popular belief that these increase cellular estrogen and aggravate estrogen dominance, they do the opposite; they balance estrogen and can decrease the damaging effects of synthetic estrogens on tissues.

Phytoestrogens:

- mimic the beneficial effects of estrogen
- block the harmful effects of high estrogen levels
- protect the body against the harmful effects of xenoestrogens
- are high in antioxidants that protect against cancer
- reduce the incidence of breast, prostate, skin and bowel cancer
- reduce cholesterol levels
- reduce the incidence of heart disease and diabetes
- help symptoms of menopause such as hot flashes, night sweats and breast tenderness
- improve symptoms of estrogen dominance
- help maintain healthy skin
- decrease bone loss

They also have an impact on decreasing mortality in women who have previously had breast cancer. Soybeans are high in phytoestrogens; however, it is important to eat only organic soy as soy is heavily sprayed with pesticides, many of which breakdown to form estrogenic fragments. Many legumes, fruits, vegetables, and whole grains exhibit phytoestrogenic effects. Tofu and tempeh are also excellent choices of phytoestrogens. When phytoestrogens are taken in pill form, such as soy-isoflavone supplements, they may be harmful to the body as they can stimulate the estrogen receptor. Soy bars should also be avoided for the same reason. It is important to remember to consume soy in its natural form as a whole food.

FOODS RICH IN PHYTOESTROGENS:

Broccoli, cauliflower, fennel, carrots, radishes, parsley, beets, apples, pomegranates, cherries, citrus fruits, soy beans, split peas, red beans, garbanzo beans, barley, oats, rice, wheat, rye, corn, garlic, sesame seeds, flax oil, and extra-virgin olive oil

---

Food as medicine for symptoms of perimenopause and menopause

Foods play an important role in either aggravating or alleviating the symptoms of menopause. With an understanding of the relationship between the food we eat and the symptoms we experience, we can make healthier food choices to promote well-being in midlife.

Foods to avoid:

- alcohol
- dairy
- excess coffee and tea
- white flour
- spicy foods
- red meat
- refined sugar
- excessive amounts of milk chocolate
- white rice

Foods to include:

- soy
- legumes
- green leafy vegetables
- tofu
- nuts
- brown rice
- melons
- seafood
- sardines
- flax
- berries
- root vegetables
- miso
- green tea
- water
- seeds
- cucumbers
- apples
- salmon
- eggs
- oats

If you use the divided plate technique, it can help simplify your food choices to include wholesome, phyto-nutrient and antioxidant rich foods into your diet. You will find that many of your symptoms will heal, and feelings of strength, vitality and health will be restored.

The inner relationship with food

Although it is important that we have knowledge of the good and "right" foods for midlife and beyond, we need to address a crucial question in every woman's life. With all the information available to us, and with all that we may know about right and wrong foods, why do we continue to make food choices that are bad for our health? Why does going on a diet feel stressful? Why do diets fail 97% of the time?

In the U.S., obesity among women is at an all-time high. Nutritionally vacant and toxic foods are widely sold in our stores. They make up the common food choices in women's lives. They are the easiest to find, with "fast food" being the least healthy for the body. We have normalized these familiar choices that are responsible for causing most of our diseases. Often our emotional, not physical hunger commonly influences our food choices, and therefore our health. Emotional hunger drives us to eat comfort foods high in fat and sugar. We lose our sensation of fullness and continue to eat even after we have had enough food to physically satisfy us. For example, we often eat foods high in fat and sugar when we are under stress. They give us a feeling of temporary comfort. This comfort does not last.

Our wounded feeling function cannot be soothed in extrinsic ways. Food does not heal our emotional pain.

Patty

Patty is a 38-year-old woman who came to me for weight loss. She had hypertension and was looking for a way to decrease the blood pressure medications she was taking. She felt that taking them was counterintuitive to her nature. Her blood pressure was only partially controlled on her medications and she was 100 pounds heavier than her ideal body weight. She needed guidance to lose weight and lower her blood pressure. She took my dietary advice and followed it for three months. She did not lose a single pound.

At her third monthly check-up, she confessed that she had been eating a pint of ice cream five nights a week before bed. After her family fell asleep, she would walk to the freezer, take out the ice cream, sit at the dining room table and devour it. It was her little secret and she felt a "high" during and after this ritual. The following morning, she would be consumed with shame. Her mind had been dominated by a shaming script that told her that she was "no good" "useless" and a "failure." During the day, she would attempt to follow my prescribed food plan. But by night, she would feel the tension between her unaddressed emotional needs and what she knew was good for her health. She looked forward to the "high" she could feel when she was alone with her ice cream after everyone had gone to sleep. She had been living in this way for years. She felt that she had no control over this and even felt shame as she described it.

My intervention for Patty was to ask her to follow through on her ice-cream ritual once more that evening and to bring her full awareness to it. I asked her to stand in front of the freezer, to take a deep breath and bring her awareness to what she was about to do, so as not to lose herself in anticipation of the familiar "high."

She tried this and was unable to eat the ice cream. She told me that she stood in front of the freezer and sobbed for an hour. She went to bed without ice-cream. In a moment of focused awareness, she had connected with her emotional pain that needed acknowledgement and healing. This pain had begun to awaken in her in midlife and the nightly ice cream ritual was her way of medicating it through the "high" that she experienced. She needed to become aware of this. Only then, could she make a more conscious choice to not allow her emotional pain to direct her behavior and take the steps needed to heal it. This was the beginning of her journey towards emotional healing. She lost 50 pounds in the next year and her blood pressure decreased. Not only did she bring consciousness to deeper areas of emotional pain that needed healing, she was able to successfully decrease her weight and blood pressure.

My journey

As someone who suffered from bulimia in my late teens and early twenties, I know only too well how Patty felt. For me, the bulimic ritual symbolized the binging and purging of academic material necessary to get through medical school. It was also a time where I could experience the "high" that connected me to a feeling of "control" in my life when I felt overwhelmed. It was my way of medicating this feeling. It was also the symbolic way that my psyche represented a disconnection from my authentic self, my feelings and instinct. This disconnection did not allow others to access me. They also kept me from accessing myself.

My healing came eight years after my eating disorder began. By then, I was worn out from it. My pleas for help and my attempts for being understood and comforted were not met by the people around me. Their denial about my condition prevented me from healing. This was also a time when eating disorders were just beginning to be acknowledged by the medical system. The medical culture that I was a part of was not able to accept that this kind of issue affected one of "their own." They were unable to help me. I was left to my own resources to heal myself.

I took my intention of healing my eating disorder to the mirror. One afternoon, I looked at myself and brought consciousness to what I saw in my reflection. I discovered that my self-talk was anything but positive. I felt that in order to heal, I needed to have positive thoughts and feelings towards myself. When I could not find anything positive to say, I heard a voice from deep inside instructing me to remain in front of the mirror until I accessed a positive thought. This took over an hour. It was something like, "I have beautiful eyes." I was determined to take this compliment into my heart, and to actually *feel* it. It took me an hour to align the thought of my eyes being beautiful with my feeling function. This alignment was momentary and I had to work hard to integrate it into my feelings towards myself. This process took months to accomplish. Before this, I had been unable to access any positive feelings towards who I felt I was, or how I looked.

Until then, my worth was dependent upon how well I performed. I felt that if I performed to perfection, I would be accepted and loved. In this way, I was driven to be a perfect performer. I was an "A" student, a perfectionist and a medical student at twenty years of age. On the inside, I had little contact with my real self. It had been replaced by doubt and suppressed by adapting to the conditioned behavior expected of me. My conditioning deeply wounded my feelings of self-worth.

I awakened to this at twenty five, when I began to bring consciousness to my relationship with my body and food. Simply bringing a positive thought towards myself in alignment with my feeling function was a new and healing experience. I became aware of how many self-critical and fear-based thoughts I had directed towards myself that affected my relationship with food. This was the gateway through which I began to heal my eating disorder. I had identified the thought patterns that led me to behave in unconscious ways which were harmful to my health. With this level of awareness, I could no longer identify with the neurosis that caused me to binge and purge for the illusory feeling of "control" in my life. When this awareness became integrated, kindness and self-compassion began to permeate my relationship to myself. I began to heal.

The journey for me, like for many others, is the journey back to ourselves. As we are able to find our will and evoke our consciousness in order to mitigate our unhealthy rituals with food, something deeper and heartfelt can awaken. This place of kindness and self-compassion is a place that is both unfamiliar and real. Often, we do not trust it. The voice of the self-critic is familiar. It is the voice of shame that evokes fear. After many years of practice, it has momentum and energy that disconnects us from having heart-centered and loving feelings towards ourselves. It is important to connect with these feelings if we are to heal our relationship with food. If we don't, our attempts at dieting will fail 97% of the time.

Fear and food

We need to stop trusting the critic in our head. We trust it because its script is reinforced by society. Our society values us mostly through our performance. Our self-worth is directly related to this. This form of externalization disconnects us from our real selves. Often, our family's definitions of our performance-based worth become imprinted in us. This awakens our inner-critic. Society's reinforcement of this definition reinforces the inner critic. Our self-evaluation is then actually determined by society. It is extrinsic. If we do not perform in accordance with society's expectations, we feel shame. We feel as though we are not "good enough" or have somehow failed. This is the way in which we begin to define our worth. We become vulnerable to abuse when we live with shame evoked by our inner-critic. Most women have such a loud critic in their heads that it disassociates them from their bodies.

Many of my obese patients tell me they do not look at themselves in the mirror. They lose contact with their feeling function. They feel emotionally regressed and vulnerable. Parts of their psyches feel infantile and they feel unsafe in their bodies and around others. When we were infants, we craved oral contact in order to feel connected and safe. When we feel vulnerable as adults, we also want to feel connected and safe. When we are vulnerable, our behavior is driven by our basic instincts. As infants, when we felt stressed and cried, we were fed. As adults, when we feel stressed from the shaming voice of the inner-critic, we feed ourselves. We regress into the infantile state. We begin to associate eating with stress. We lose our sense of limits and boundaries. We overeat.

My work with women to help them heal their relationship

with food also helps them heal their relationship with themselves. The emotional pressures they feel when they think about losing weight evoke their fear of failure. It is not possible to fully engage in healthy behaviors when there is fear lurking in our psyches. We need to support each other into loving ourselves enough to reduce the momentum of fear and heal our worth that we have erroneously identified with performance. We need to dismantle these conditioned feelings in order to reclaim our intrinsic worth.

Women doubt their ability to heal and reclaim their health. They doubt their ability to reframe their definitions of success and self-worth. None of us can do this work alone. We require a sisterhood of women who have gone before us and have succeeded in this difficult return to self to hold space for our process. Without this, it is difficult to build the endurance and the momentum needed for the spiritual practice of self- love.

Midlife consciousness and our relationship to food

As we explore the midlife journey and its powerful and terrifying process of coming into our truth and intrinsic power, we can be transformed for the better. Even though the voices of shame may remain, through our awareness they will weaken and lose momentum. The voices of self-compassion and understanding will replace them. As we heal our behaviors in relationship to food, we can begin to heal our primal wounds, as well as, our separation from our real selves.

Our healing can begin when we bring consciousness to our rituals of eating; at first for moments and then for longer, until a new pattern of conscious eating emerges. If a woman diets with the intention of annihilating her voices of shame, or with the fear of failing, she cannot achieve her goals. Only through becoming conscious and engaging patience and self-compassion can the process of healing and repair succeed. The shaming critic in a woman's head does not allow for self-care. Loving behavior is in contrast to the inner-critic's shaming directives. If she is unaware, the inner-critic can control her relationship with herself. It can dominate her inner-world. The inner-critic goes dormant periodically, and often rises up again to sabotage attempts at self-empowerment and health, when she begins to make positive changes. She must keep moving forward and inward towards her real self in order to build new momentum, despite difficulties or even occasional failures. Every failure is a lesson learned that can serve to deepen her consciousness. This is necessary for self-healing. It is important for us to remind each other of this during the moments of struggle on this difficult yet healing journey towards emotional and physical health.

Our society normalizes our critical and self-sabotaging behavior. Our society itself is in paradox. On the one hand, we are experiencing a crisis of obesity and on the other hand, clothing companies have expanded their sizes to accommodate bigger bodies. This is a subtle yet illusory way of hiding reality from consumers. A size 10 today is larger than it was five years ago. The clothing industry is attempting to give women the *illusion* of being a smaller size than they really are. This perpetuates illusions and untruths about our bodies that we need to uncover and dismantle.

A commitment to a better and healthier relationship with food can include some of the following steps:

- Bring consciousness to a feeling of fullness while eating.

- Learn the language of the inner-critic and behave in ways that are contrary to its orders for self-shaming and abuse. These behaviors can lessen the control that the inner-critic has on promoting unhealthy behaviors.

- Make a commitment to yourself witnessed by a trusted friend who can remind you of your progress when the momentum of the inner-critics script takes over, attempting to sabotage forward movement.

- Invest in personal growth through psychotherapy in order to transform your relationship to yourself into one that supports self-care and authenticity.

There are many ways to reclaim our health through our relationship with food. We each need to find our own unique path and practice it. Despite setbacks along the way, we need to stay on the path that is conscious and stay open to learning and seeking. Staying on the path is more important than failing a hundred times. This builds the endurance contained in the archetypes of the Warrior and Heroine and brings women into connection with themselves and their intrinsic worth. Unless we become conscious of our inner dialogues, they will continue to direct our behaviors and keep us entranced and disconnected from our bodies.

This process requires both courage and consciousness. It may be difficult at first, but I promise you that it will be worth the effort invested when you can view yourself through an intrinsic lens of worth that is aligned with your feeling function. Living from self-compassion is a spiritual path. Developing a healthy relationship with food can heal our many levels of wounding. It can also heal our wounded relationship with nature and bring joy and vitality to the time we spend within our families and communities. Food can become a form of art and "medicine" in our culture. It is imperative for us to reintegrate this lost art into our culture for our collective healing.

5

The Four Body System

Integrative medicine makes sense. People are innately connected to this concept because it is inclusive and connective. It makes sense to utilize disciplines that have been time tested over thousands of years and have worked for millions of people before traditional medicine emerged. Creating a system of health care that is truly integrative, however, requires more than just placing multidisciplinary modalities together under one roof. It requires practicing medicine from an open system that works from many levels in contrast to a closed system that focuses only on physical pathology (the study and diagnosis of disease). This requires us to expand our view of health and illness through more than just the physically oriented framework. This is the only way we can effectively utilize the techniques of ancient disciplines which have healed many illnesses with far greater success than the traditional medical model. It involves engaging a new and expanded lens that can identify the levels from which illness emerges.

The current framework of integrative medicine in health care is incomplete. From its perspective, "mind-body" medicine is the more complete approach to health and illness. However, the "mind-body" connection is too limited for healing the foundational roots of illness. The mind is limited. It adapts in order to help us survive. Its focus is narrow. In recent years, we have discovered our ability to manipulate biology by changing the way we project our mind towards circumstances that cause us discomfort. We try to replace our negative thinking with positive thinking in order to help alleviate our symptoms and manipulate our physiology. We know through science that the "mind" is in the body. We have discovered that neurotransmitters and receptors that affect our mood, thinking and physical health are present throughout our body, and this scientifically validates mind-body medicine. However, the manipulation of the body with the mind is limited in what it can do to *truly* heal and restore balance at deeper levels. In the nineties, we were taught to use positive thinking and visualizations to produce "good" chemicals in the brain and body in order to heal. Early in my career, I utilized this framework, but found it limited for true healing in several ways:

1. We cannot fool ourselves into thinking what we don't feel. If we feel sad due to a life event or experience that causes us grief or anger, positive *thinking* cannot change our *feelings*. We will still have to process our feelings in order to return to a state of balance. Our feelings will override any attempts we may make to change them through thinking. We can try to think positively, and this may work for a while, but eventually, our real feelings will surface. Sometimes they present as emotional symptoms and sometimes as physical symptoms. This occurs due to the emotional pressure that can build from the invalidation of our feeling function in favor of thinking. For example, heart attacks are more common on Monday mornings at 9 a.m. when people begin their work week. This is thought to be a result of an increase in stress hormones that are affected by feelings in the Emotional body that activate coronary spasm. If these feelings are processed and the causes of work stress are addressed, this can lower the level of stress hormones produced by the adrenals and reduce the risk of heart attacks on Monday mornings. No amount of positive thinking can lower this risk. It can only be lowered by addressing the feeling function.

2. When life experiences cause us to become fearful, mind-body medicine would suggest that we can talk ourselves out of fear. This

endangers the validity of our fearful feelings. Fear is the body's attempt to protect us but sometimes it can become chronic and this can damage our health. Fear warns us that danger is near. In circumstances where fear may become chronic, such as in toxic working conditions or in toxic relationships, it may manifest as symptoms of anxiety or depression. If we believe then that we can heal these symptoms by thinking positively and are unable to, we may feel as though we have somehow failed in not being able to assert our minds over our bodies. This can activate our inner-critic. The conditions that cause chronic fear need to be evaluated and processed.

3. "Mind-body" solutions have the danger of evoking *shame* in people who have sensitive feeling function. They are often unable to override their feelings with positive thinking.

Sensitive people or "sensitives" relate to life kinesthetically. They process information and life experiences through their senses, not through their minds. For example, when they are in a crowd they often feel agitated. This is because when they are around others, "sensitives" feel the energy of others. When they process information or have memories, they *feel* them rather than think about them. Their feeling function is more engaged in processing life than their thinking function. Since our culture values thinking over feeling, "sensitives" have a difficult time feeling validated. They feel out of place in a society that values mind over feelings and sometimes think that they are ill due to their intense feeling state.

Feeling function becomes more pronounced in midlife as a woman's physiology begins to change. Not being able to manipulate the body with the mind or change negative feelings with positive thinking, sets a midlife woman up for feeling shame and inadequacy in her inability to have control over the intensity of her feeling function. Healing is not deep enough through "mind-body" approaches if feeling function and emotional processes are not addressed and validated.

4. When we experience life events, we carry their memories and energy in our "energy fields." For the past 100 years, our culture has not had a framework to include, acknowledge or understand the energetic aspects of our body. These neglected aspects are often the causal levels that impact our health at emotional, mental and physical levels. We ignore these aspects of ourselves due to the lack of framework present in our society, and often miss the opportunity to heal imbalances at these levels. The energy field also carries memories from our life histories. This field is not able to heal with mental or physical manipulation. It is much deeper and more abstract than mental or physical states. It has to be addressed with healing techniques that can diagnose energetic imbalances and correct their *manifestations* in the other levels of the body. The imbalances at energetic levels manifest as symptoms in other levels.

The two "bodies" we focus on in our medical model are the *Physical body* and the *Mental body*. We need to open our current paradigm to accommodate two other bodies, the *Emotional body*, the level directly related to our feeling function, and the *Energy body*, the level from where both illnesses and true health emerge. These bodies are directly affected by our life experiences, our thinking and our feeling function. These profoundly affect our physiology and our ability to *truly* heal.

Clearly, we need a framework to understand ourselves beyond the "mind-body" framework; one that includes the *Emotional and Energy bodies*. We have focused only on the "mind-body" for the past two decades, and have not gone beyond it. Science has investigated ways the mind can heal the body. The danger of approaching our lives and our health from this limited "mind-body" framework within the closed system of medicine reinforces our attempts to dominate and manipulate the body with the mind. Our culture engages the concept of mind *over* matter. This concept places us in a mode of conquest where we attempt to conquer illnesses with the power of the mind. This framework is limited and limiting and does not offer us intrinsic health. Its limitations reinforce our feelings of powerlessness and failure if we are unable to fulfill its goals.

Cartesian theory

In traditional medicine, the focus on the Physical body and its clinical analysis is based on reductionism. The body is broken down into its component parts in order to search for the physical causes of its symptoms. This narrows the focus to fix only the physical level without accounting for the emotional or energetic levels. In this way, the power and effect of other levels is negated in favor of fixing physical symptoms. Although the emotional and energetic aspects of the body are not physically visible, they have powerful effects on the Physical body. They cannot be seen, but they are felt. In working from a physically focused Cartesian framework, the connection to the emotional and energetic aspects of patients is compromised. Due to the limits of this paradigm, physicians lose sight of wholeness and process, both important qualities of the Feminine Principle. They also lose sight of the impact of the Emotional and Energy bodies. It is possible for us to maintain our Cartesian approach while including deeper levels of cause, while we analyze their role in the manifestation of illness and health. In their absence, medical analysis often remains incomplete and limits the patient's ability to truly heal.

The art of healing

Healing is the work of connection and the art of relationship. A healer needs good listening skills. The listening required for healing needs to occur through the ears, the eyes and the heart. The levels that the heart engages are not accessible to the mind. The mind engages through analysis. Within the mind, component parts seem manageable. All that is needed is expertise and mastery in order to control and fix. For the patient, this feels disconnected and sterile.

A physician's heart is as important to the patient as mind and expertise. The heart holds space and is open to possibilities. It bears witness. It validates and loves. The energy of love and presence sometimes does more for healing than mastery and expertise that are engaged in uncovering and fixing pathology. Patients are fearful. Fear is the main emotion they feel in relationship to physicians, even when all is well. They worry that expertise will uncover problems within their bodies. Physicians must be sensitive to this. There is a term in medicine known as "white-coat hypertension." This is an elevation of blood pressure that results from the fear of being in a physician's office. Physicians need to be sensitive to the fear that patients carry when they come to see them. With this awareness, they can better hold an empathic and understanding space which can help their patients heal more effectively. They must be able hold space for their patient's process and offer them validation. There can be no healing without the exploration of process and "fixing" alone is inadequate to address the depth of the patient's needs.

The female patient

For the midlife woman, the health care practitioner's capacity to evoke healing and wholeness is critical for her healing and transformation. A woman can keenly sense if the practitioner is connected to their heart and feeling function. If there is no contact from this place, she has difficulty trusting the expertise offered. The patient's intuition and feelings also render her suspicious and skeptical of the expert, as she needs connection with both the physician's expertise and empathy. Unfortunately, many women second-guess their need for both. Their continued fear and lack of resonance with the physician is a sign that something essential is missing in their relationship. But they feel limited in their options. They are fearful and are looking for relief from the discomfort of their symptoms. When they settle for expertise at the cost of connection they invalidate their real needs. In addition, this "settling for" contributes to the health care system's continued absence of heart centered focus.

This is the dilemma many midlife women face after multiple encounters with physicians who have analyzed their symptoms and reduced them to merely a physiological deficiency of estrogen. The expert medical solution to their symptoms has often been synthetic hormone replacement and antidepressants, with little or no attention to process. Women are looking for a framework that helps them understand and validate their process. They lose trust in expertise-oriented physicians who do not create a safe space for their needs.

The cost of emotional neglect

We have side-stepped our feeling function for the sake of being accepted by a culture that has put it on the back burner. The Emotional body contains our feeling function. Our emotions are the closest contact that we have with our souls. As a culture, have been raised to undermine this aspect of ourselves and are paying deeply for this. Our repressed and covered over feelings build pressure in our Emotional bodies until they spill over as "dis-ease." Any feeling that is repressed will rise up in another way to release its pressure. Denial and repression of our feelings are bad for our health. It is our sacred work to reawaken our relationship with our souls through understanding and validating our feelings by releasing the energy we have repressed within for the first half of our lives. Most of us have adapted to society and its invalidation of our feelings by repressing them. The biological shift in our hormones manifests our need for cleansing these patterns. Initially, as intense feelings emerge, we may feel as though we are losing emotional ground. But as we understand the ways in which we have denied our needs in order to comply with society's expectations, we can understand the intensity contained in the Emotional body. Since our feelings were often not validated, we need support from others in addition to a framework through which we can understand our body's need for emotional release. We need to remember that our feelings are never wrong.

This process is a difficult one. It is often preceded by an amorphous rage that many women feel that they may direct towards their spouses and/or children, those to whom they have given over of themselves in a caretaking role for most of their adult lives. The learned and imprinted patterns they have behaved from while denying their own needs in favor of others are no longer acceptable and this history of self-denial emerges through feelings of deep rage. Many midlife women do not understand this process and are frightened by it. They feel shame at emoting towards their spouses and children for even little requests asked of them. Their families are perplexed and bewildered by this rage and it creates stress in family systems. Sometimes everyone connected with the transitioning woman finds themselves walking on eggshells around her.

Mary

Mary is a 39-year-old woman who came to see me for symptoms of fatigue and heavy menstrual bleeding. She felt stressed after taking on an in-home child care position to babysit three children below the ages of four, in addition to caregiving her own three children. She did this to help her family's finances after her husband lost his job. Within a month of doing this, she found herself losing patience with her own children and snapping at them frequently. In addition, she was not able to express kindness to the children she was care-giving, and felt anger towards them for her feelings of depletion. She felt shame around the feelings of rage she had towards her children, and resentment towards the children she was care-giving. She said she felt like a "bad mother and wife," unable to help her family in a time of need.

It was clear from her heavy periods that her progesterone levels were dropping. She was also feeling intensity in her Emotional body that she did not understand. She began to realize that she only felt this way in the areas of her life where she believed she was expected to compromise her personal limits for social duty.

While listening to her story, I asked who she thought was responsible for knowing her limits and her boundaries. She acknowledged that it was hers. She realized that she projected this responsibility onto her husband and expected him to advocate for her to not continue offering childcare. Her husband had just found new employment and was adjusting to new work hours and the learning curve of a new job. He was under stress himself. She felt ashamed for admitting that the responsibilities she had taken on with child care overwhelmed her and disrupted the balance in her life. All her attempts at logical and positive thinking had failed.

As she uncovered her pattern of self-sacrifice at the cost of her sovereignty and gained awareness of her tendency to override her limits for the sake of "duty," she understood that her Emotional body was responding to her appropriately. She was conditioned not to speak her truth and to compromise it in favor of what she thought was expected. She had learned to override her limits for the sake of others. She had been conditioned to do this by her family of origin and by society. She realized that overriding her instinctive cues with cultural expectations as a dutiful wife and mother was toxic to her body. Her emotions were reacting from rage towards the patterns of her own conditioned behavior that caused her to deny her needs. She realized that obeying her limits through acts of self-care was the most powerful gift she could offer herself and her family as well as the children she was resentfully babysitting. She quit her job as an in-home daycare provider. She became aware of the ways in which her intuition informed her about her personal limits through intense feelings that arose within her when they were compromised. Since then, she is much happier, and so is her family.

The importance of aligning with feeling function

These are the crucial issues of our time, and in midlife, we are called to reframe and expand our personal paradigms. Our sacred task is to heal the deep wounds of self-neglect that arise in midlife through our feeling function. We need to dispel the idea of "getting over" intense feelings of grief, rage and sadness, and rather learn how to work with them respectfully. Without this, we can never fully heal. An increase in impotence and infertility in our society, although heavily influenced by our polluted environment, is symbolic of this rupture in feeling function. Deep feelings are prerequisites for erotic and vivacious creativity. Without them, the energy of the soul is dimmed and fertility is thwarted. Despite our ability to restore sexual function with the use of medications, and become pregnant with the use of synthetic hormones, our souls continue to hunger for erotic and the animated feelings, the feelings that evoke creativity. Drugs can never offer us this and neither can the framework of "mind over body." If we attempt to fix our problems of diminished feeling function only at the physical level and expect our mind to "get over" our emotions, we will remain unhealed at core levels. We often fool ourselves into thinking that we have healed when we use medications to suppress our emotions and mistake symptomatic cure for core healing. In this manner we remain collectively wounded at both emotional and cultural levels.

Jungian author and analyst, Robert Johnson states that *the cultural masculine and feminine kill the natural masculine and feminine. Nature responds by making the cultural man and woman impotent.* I believe he means that the cultural definitions of masculine and feminine have replaced what we intuitively know as the healthy masculine and feminine. In order for our fertile nature to unfold, we must behave in ways that engage our healthy masculine and feminine energies. Without addressing the impact that our obedience to societal expectations has on impotence and infertility, we will be unable to find real solutions to these growing challenges.

The relationship of the Four Bodies

Over the years, I have worked with thousands of patients and have gained an awareness of how trauma, shock and bewilderment, all common experiences in life, deeply affect our health. We do not pay much attention to the levels that need understanding and release for *true* healing. Our focus is usually in the form of mental and physical interventions. As a result, we only partially heal from trauma. The underlying energy system that holds the shock and memory of our experiences is not addressed. Its healing plays an integral role for our *true* healing and recovery.

For example, if someone is in a car accident, the shock and trauma that accompany this event can get stuck at multiple levels of the body. As people heal the physical injury caused by the accident, they may begin to experience anxiety. The trauma of an accident can manifest in time as chronic anxiety. People are perplexed by this feeling, especially if their physical trauma has healed. They describe the anxiety as tightness or agitation in their bodies. They feel it as a constriction or an ache that is accompanied by feelings of being overwhelmed. When they experience this, they do not feel safe in their skins. Their anxiety usually has a life of its own. They find their bodies becoming tense when they pass the location of the accident, and find themselves replaying the accident in their minds. They may develop insomnia as a result of this repetitive recapitulation. They may experience palpitations, or feelings of emotional paralysis and irritability. They may attempt to medicate their anxiety with prescription drugs or alcohol in order to control these feelings that randomly ebb and flow. Their anxiety often leads them to the emergency room or their doctor's office if it becomes chronic. Their doctors may medicate them to suppress the anxiety. The medications may have side effects that add to their lack of well-being. They fear that they may have developed an anxiety disorder as a result of the accident.

When we expand the medical framework beyond the Physical body to include the Energy and Emotional bodies, this can help us to understand the levels that are impacted by trauma that manifest symptoms of both physical pain and anxiety. We can also gain insight about how this can lead to self-medicating behaviors for symptomatic relief. The cause of these symptoms lies deep in the Energy body, where the memories of trauma and shock that accompanied the accident reside. Unless this level is addressed, and the trauma is released, there is a risk of it getting stuck and having it manifest as anxiety. The patient in this instance would be *incorrectly* labeled with an anxiety disorder. What she needs is the understanding that her anxiety is a manifestation of the trauma that accompanied the accident that is held in her Energy body. If she is labeled and medicated, the *cause* of the anxiety would not be addressed; only its *manifestation* would be medicated.

A view of the Four Body System

1. The Physical body is the *densest* of the four bodies and where physical symptoms manifest. This is the main area of focus by the framework of traditional medicine.

2. The Mental body is *less dense* than the Physical body. It manifests symptoms of imbalance through behaviors that indicate that it requires attention and process. This is the area of focus by the fields of psychiatry and psychology.

3. The Emotional body, the area of feeling function, is even *less dense* than the Mental body. This is where and 'gut' or intuitive feelings are felt. This is where feelings of anxiety and depression, grief and rage arise. This is an area that is denied and neglected by our cultural and medical framework. It has a significant influence on the health of the Physical and Mental bodies. The fields of psychiatry and psychology address the body physically with medications

and mentally, with behavior modification and psychotherapy. Physically based approaches such as medications, provide symptom management for manifestations at the mental level, but do not truly heal them. The Emotional body requires an integrative approach through a variety of therapies including psychotherapy and energy work that can balance it for *true* healing.

4. The Energy body is the *least dense* body, but it affects the health of all of the other bodies. This is the area where *causes* of illness emerge and where it's healing can affect the *true* healing of the Emotional, Mental and Physical bodies. The disciplines of flower essence therapy, homeopathy, breath work, Reiki and Traditional Chinese medicine all impact and influence the health of the Energy body (figure 4).

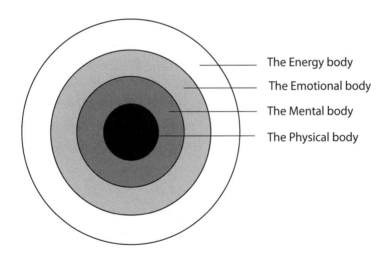

The Energy body

The Emotional body

The Mental body

The Physical body

Figure 4: The Four Body System

We are all aware of the ways that our Physical and Mental bodies manifest illness. This is the popular framework accepted by society and the medical system. My goal is to offer a conceptual understanding of the Energy and Emotional bodies with methods to balance and heal them. This will help clarify where illness and health emerge from and how one can heal at these levels of cause. It is important for us to expand our definition of health to accommodate these bodies in order for *true* healing to occur.

The Energy body

The Energy body is the largest and most subtle container that surrounds and houses the Physical body. The Energy body has four main components:

1. the electrical system
2. the constitutional system
3. the meridians or energy lines
4. the subtle body

The electrical system

The electrical system is the part of the Energy body that regulates and affects the heart rhythm, nervous system and muscles. We can measure the electrical activity of these three systems with diagnostic medical tools. We can measure the heart rhythms with an electrocardiogram (EKG), nerve impulses with an electroencephalogram (EEG), and the electrical activity of muscles with an electromyogram (EMG). The electrical system is both electrical and magnetic. Although this part of the body is invisible, it has a profound impact on the heart rhythms, the nervous system (and its sensitivity and conductivity), and neuromuscular junctions that are present in muscles. They all conduct electricity and are impacted by aberrations in the electrical system. The electrical system creates the electromagnetic field surrounding the Physical body. This field is up to eight feet in diameter around the Physical body. Its activity can be measured by a galvanometer, a device used to measure electrical currents. The electrical system is affected by trauma, shock and violence, as well as, love and happiness.

The Institute of HeartMath in California has shown that when one is in a state of stress, the electrical activity of the heart changes to a rhythm that indicates the signals flowing through the nervous system as out of sync and disordered. This rhythm can be measured through a technique called *heart rate variability analysis*. There is a specific time and space between each heartbeat. The Institute of HeartMath has found that an increased variability between heartbeats correlates with a greater resilience of the heart, especially when one is under stress. In other words, the increased variation in time and space between each heart beat indicates an increase in the heart's resilience, and a reduction in cardiac risk. It is likened to a loose rubber band as compared to one that is tightly stretched. The one that is loose has a greater degree of elasticity, variability or resilience than one that is tight and does not have as much elasticity, variability or resilience. A decrease in variability offers the heart less flexibility and resilience, increasing cardiac risk. It is much easier for a tight rubber band to snap than a loose one. The highly variable or low risk rhythm looks like a smooth sine wave and the less variable or high risk rhythm looks jagged and linear (figure 5).

In the first graph in figure 5, under the influence of the emotions of frustration and anger, the beat to beat variability is short and the heart rate variability shows a jagged appearance. In the second graph, under the influence of the emotion of sincere appreciation, the heart rate variability graph shows a larger and more regular rhythm called a sine wave. It is smooth and cyclic. Anger causes the heart to have erratic activity and appreciation causes its electrical activity to become more synchronized. This demonstrates that emotions affect the electrical activity of the heart.

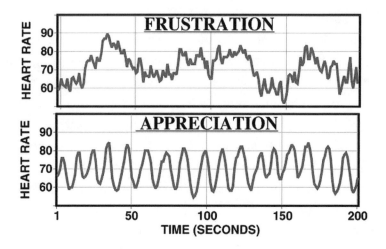

Figure 5: Heart rate variability graphs
(Reprinted with written permission—Institute of HeartMath ©1998, 2011)

This is one example of the impact that the Energy and Emotional bodies have on the Physical body. The energetic properties of feelings and emotions have direct effects on health in both negative and positive ways. The electrical system responds to feelings. These feelings impact the Physical body in ways that can be measured through analyzing the heart rate variability. This has a direct correlation with cardiac risk. By becoming more aware of the correlations between feelings and health, we can improve our emotional and physical health in ways that prescription drugs cannot. By By understanding the effect that our feelings have on our physiology, we can learn to respond to situations in more balanced ways that can preserve the health of our electrical system.

Energy memory

The Energy body has the capacity to remember every experience ever encountered. Traumatic memories trapped in this body can impact the electrical activity of the heart. The Energy body remembers experiences even without conscious memory of them. It does not have the ability to filter out negative memories. There are times it remembers what we don't, and we wonder why we feel what we do. It is not uncommon for us to feel emotional agitation during the anniversary of a birth, death, divorce, accident or significant event from the past. It is the memory stored in the Energy body that reminds us of the event due to its recall of a specific time in our biography. For example, we may find ourselves agitated or sad for no obvious reason and when we realize it is associated with the anniversary of an event from the past, we can provide ourselves with needed self-care and self-support. The nature of the event and the way it was experienced in the past, effects our emotions in the present. These memories are held in the Energy body.

Flower essence therapy
There is a discipline unfamiliar to traditional medicine which many alternative healers utilize due to its profound impact on the electrical system. It involves a pharmacy of remedies called "flower essences." Flower essence therapy was established by Dr. Edward Bach. His healing framework described illness as "a force with the potential to facilitate the process required in dealing with the spiritual and psychological issues neglected before the illness manifested." He believed that illness was one way that destiny tried to help us deepen and evolve. He noticed relationships between different personalities and the types of illnesses they manifested. He also found that certain flowers and plants could support and nurture the Energy body in ways that could balance and stabilize the Energy body of the person experiencing the illness.

Dr. Bach saw flowers as "receptors for the soul gestures of the cosmos." When a flower is placed in water in sunlight, he found the water would incorporate the energetic essence of the flower. When ingested, it could shift the emotional and energetic patterns of the person ingesting it and make their patterns more flexible. This would sometimes lead to emotional healing and also impact physical illness in positive ways. The essence could in fact, assist the person to fortify their system against trauma, which made them vulnerable, and even strengthen them to be able to release the trauma held in the Energy body.

We can apply this framework to the case of the accident described previously that resulted in anxiety, insomnia and repetitive thoughts. These are all manifestations of shock and trauma resulting from the accident. These symptoms can be released to a large degree by taking a flower essence called Star of Bethlehem, which is prescribed specifically for trauma. The body is able to heal more quickly at all levels, when the associated mental and emotional symptoms due to trauma are released.

Dr. Bach observed that the plant known as Star of Bethlehem grew in moderately harsh environments. Its flower contained properties of hardiness and when given to those in vulnerable states, they incorporated its properties of hardiness and resilience. When he prepared this essence by his extraction methods and gave it to people that had experienced traumatic events, they were able to heal the anxiety associated with the traumatic memories trapped in the Energy body. This is one example of how flower essence therapy works. Dr. Bach created a pharmacy of essences which correlated the healing characteristics of plants and flowers with symptom relief in humans and animals. This pharmacy has the ability to heal many imbalances in the Energy body that manifest as symptoms in the Mental and Physical bodies. Since these essences work at subtle levels, they must be taken regularly for a prolonged periods of time, under the guidance of a flower essence practitioner in order for them to be most effective.

When we expand our framework of health to include an understanding of the impact that the Energy body has on our state of well-being, we can understand how the limited framework of traditional medicine can lead to overuse pharmaceuticals for symptomatic relief without healing the underlying causes that may lie in the Energy body. When issues at the energetic level are not addressed, they "spill over" into the Emotional, Mental and Physical bodies as symptoms. Energy cannot be created or destroyed. It simply changes form. An imbalanced or traumatized Energy body can directly impact the Physical and Mental bodies. When flooded with trauma, it can lead to illnesses resulting from stress hormones. We often see this in people with Post-Traumatic-Stress-Disorder or PTSD. The toxic effects of stress hormones can cause physical conditions such as ulcers, esophageal reflux, headaches, colitis, muscle pain, fibromyalgia, chronic fatigue, insomnia, dizziness, and vertigo to name only a few. Obesity can be an eventual manifestation of trauma if the patient overeats to medicate the anxiety caused by the trauma present in the Energy body. Obesity, alone, can lead to a myriad of diseases such as diabetes, heart disease, strokes, and hypertension.

The impact of the electrical system's state of balance and imbalance plays a significant role in the health of our Energy, Emotional and Mental bodies. When addressed through flower essence therapy, it can sometimes alleviate the most subtle imbalances that may be causative factors in anxiety that manifest in the Mental body, but have their roots in the electrical system.

The car accident example demonstrates the power of flower essence therapy. Interventions at this level help realign the electrical system when it leads to mental symptoms resulting from trauma. Understanding the process at this level can help us seek practitioners who are skilled in this form of therapy and can recommend combinations of flower essences that can precisely address the symptoms resulting from emotional and energetic imbalances. This can support the Energy body in the same way as traditional medical and psychological interventions can support manifestations at denser levels of the Mental and Physical bodies.

The constitutional system

Classical homeopathy is a discipline that restores constitutional balance to the Energy body by correcting chronic and sometimes acute aggravations of symptoms that can occur when the system becomes imbalanced from stress. The constitutional system is the part of the Energy body that is responsible for feelings of "intrinsic stability" in relationship to life circumstances.

As humans, we adapt to stress on a daily basis. Most of our adaptations are mediated by responses and compensations for survival. For example, we may compensate for our fear of failure by overworking or through our drive for perfectionism. This may promote behaviors that we term "workaholic." Through these behaviors, we may neglect our boundaries and limits. These behaviors are compensations that can deplete us. We can try to repair our behaviors through psychotherapy and behavior modification, but unless the underlying condition—our fear of failure, is addressed, it will often surface from our Energy body and drive us to behave in compensatory ways. Over time, this can lead to adrenal stress and many physical symptoms may manifest with precision directed by our constitutional makeup. Our constitution is deeply impacted by our adaptations to stress. It can become imbalanced over time, resulting in chronic symptoms that call for constitutional healing.

Homeopathy is a 200-year-old system of healing, and its underlying philosophy restores energetic balance to a person's constitution. *Homeo* means "same or similar" and *pathy* means "disease." Derived from the plant, mineral and animal kingdoms, homeopathic remedies are capable of producing mild symptoms in healthy people, yet also help to resolve those same symptoms in people who are sick.

The homeopathic approach begins with the understanding that a person is an integrated whole and in response to the challenges of life, is engaged in an ongoing dynamic effort to maintain balance. Under normal circumstances one responds to and "rebounds" from various stresses, hopefully a stronger and wiser person. However, when challenges are too strong or too prolonged, one can become stuck in a dysfunctional stress response. The manifested symptoms are defined as disease. Rather than suppressing the symptoms created by the stress response, the homeopathic remedy works to cue the person's system as to how one's adaptation are unhealthy, or how the manner in which a person adapts to stress imbalances their constitution. This, in turn, provokes a healing reaction in the Energy body.

Based on the person's history (which unfolds during a two-hour interview), the certified classical homeopath works to understand the unique individuality and the state of imbalance present in the patient's constitution. A very specific remedy is then chosen which amplifies the internal awareness or the body's "inner wisdom." According to homeopathy, the body's inner wisdom will recognize the state that resulted in "dis-ease" when the correct remedy is introduced into the body. This in turn, provokes a deep and integrated self-healing reaction on physical, mental and emotional levels. By using this precise approach, homeopathy supports the person's own innate healing potential, resulting in a safe and natural return to health.

Arlene

Arlene is a 55-year-old woman who came to me with complaints of severe and chronic asthma and recurrent panic attacks for 10 years. These symptoms began soon after she divorced her abusive husband of twenty years. During her marriage, she lived from a fight-or-flight response pattern, adapting to the abuse with the methods she was raised with from her family of origin. After she left her husband and felt physically safe, she began to have panic attacks which were treated with three different medications by her traditional medical doctors. In addition, she was taking four medications in an attempt to prevent asthma attacks which brought her to the emergency room a couple times a year. She had been on multiple medications for many years. She came to me seeking a "cure" for her symptoms as they were taking a toll on her quality of life and her finances.

After interviewing her about the nature of her attacks and the feelings surrounding her panic, it was clear to me that her adaptations had taken a toll on her constitutional balance. Since she did not have to adapt to survival issues around abuse any longer due to her changed environment, she did not understand why she continued to have the symptoms that she did.

I referred Arlene to a certified classical homeopath. After an extensive interview, the remedy that the homeopath selected was one derived from the willow tree. Arlene had survived abuse over a prolonged period of time by creating an "energetic wall" that offered her the feeling of "safety." It had resulted in characteristics of inflexibility in her nature that she had developed as a reaction to abuse. She developed this wall unconsciously through her energetic patterns in order to feel safe around abuse. This also manifested in dynamics she had in other relationships. For example, if someone offered her constructive criticism, her "energetic wall" would go up and she would get defensive and reactive. If someone tried to connect with her in relationship, she would push them away with her "energetic wall" as she would feel afraid that she would be mistreated in the relationship. After the chronic stress passed with her divorce, she no longer needed this "energetic wall" to feel safe. But after years, this had become her adapted pattern for survival. It was causing her to continue to react to even minor stressors from the exaggerated patterns of inflexibility conditioned by years of abuse. It had manifested in symptoms of severe anxiety and asthma. The remedy which contained the energy of the willow tree was more like her innate balanced constitution. This remedy resonated with her unadapted state of flexibility and reawakened it in her Energy body, restoring balance to it. It helped her Energy body revert back to this flexible state which was characteristic of her state of constitutional health. Within six weeks of taking the willow remedy, Arlene's asthma healed and her panic improved so dramatically that she was weaned off her medications within a relatively short period of time.

She no longer visited the emergency room for asthma attacks. I taught her about the benefits of anti-inflammatory foods to prevent her asthma from being activated from the physical level. She had been eating inflammatory foods in order to comfort her anxiety, which also activated her asthma. She changed her diet to one consisting of whole foods and began taking moderate doses Omega-3. Within six months, her asthma fully healed without recurrence with this combination of therapies. After eight years of follow-up, I am happy to report she has not had a single panic or asthma attack.

She was able to shift out of the inflexible state of survival into a flexible state of constitutional balance offered by the remedy from the willow tree. Providing the homeopathic history also brought a sense of awareness to her adapted state. With this awareness, she was able to manage her anxiety in healthier ways when it became activated under stress. Now when her survival patterns arise and her anxiety surfaces her awareness of its origins motivates her to treat herself with self-compassion. She is able to consistently behave in ways that offer her resilience and a rapid recovery from her symptoms.

As I broadened my perceptual framework for evaluating chronic symptoms that my traditional tool box could only palliate, I began to gain a perspective of health and illness that included an awareness of how symptoms can manifest as a result of an imbalanced constitution. Adapted and conditioned behaviors can often imbalance one's state of intrinsic constitutional balance. This imbalance can then manifest as physical and mental symptoms.

We adapt in order to survive. Survival is the basic instinct that keeps us alive under threat. Even when the threat is minor, our brains are programmed to activate the fight-or-flight response for survival. Fear activates the stress response. It can exaggerate our reactions to stressors by distorting our perceptions and exaggerating the reactions we have learned through our imprinting. If our parents were frequently fearful or anxious, we may have been imprinted with the perception that we are not safe in the world. The constitutional imbalances that result from adaptations like these are deep, and expressed with precision in our biology. In this manner, our biographies have a profound impact on our adaptations to stress. These adaptations can cause constitutional imbalances that manifest as chronic mental and physical symptoms. In our traditional medical system, this perspective is not included in differential diagnosis or therapeutic interventions. These are powerful and important aspects of health that have a significant impact on how we feel and how we heal. When physicians begin to include this perspective in their framework of diagnosis and treatment, it can have profound effects on both patients' abilities to both heal in addition to improving their responses to traditional medical treatments.

It is important that only credentialed homeopaths be engaged, those with thousands of hours of clinical training and experience, and certified through the Medical Society of Homeopathy. Not all homeopaths are trained in classical homeopathy, which addresses and heals constitutional imbalances. Very few are trained and experienced enough to be effective in helping chronic symptoms. Discernment is needed to differentiate credible homeopaths from "pop" healers who practice homeopathy without extensive training. A homeopath that is not skilled and credentialed can harm a chronically ill patient if the high standards of classical homeopathy are not practiced. Many claim credentialing, but receive it through internet courses, and do not have the clinical experience necessary for *healing*. They may use homeopathic remedies to merely palliate symptoms, but this does not lead to constitutional healing. The art of this discipline is as important as its technique.

We need to establish high standards of care for non-traditional practitioners in order to keep patients safe. We need to employ instinct and logic as well as self-responsibility, until high standards are established, for safe and effective healing. Too often, people gravitate towards less than adequately trained non-traditional practitioners due to their disappointment with the traditional medical system, and they do not discern for quality care. It is important to stay aware of this danger in selecting a practitioner for restoring health.

The subtle body

The subtle body within the energy system consists of two main components:

   1. the breath
   2. the chakra system

The breath

Throughout the history of the human race, there has been an awareness of the influence that breathing has on health. Breathing is integral to the discipline of yoga, where the breath is used to oxygenate muscles and create a connection with consciousness. Yoga is a discipline that links the mind, body and subtle body. Breath is the connector of all three. It is cyclic like nature. It ebbs and flows. When we inhale, we oxygenate the body; when we exhale, we detoxify it. This cycle of inhalation and exhalation is life sustaining. If it is interrupted for too long, life itself is threatened. Life energy is dependent upon breath.

When we are stressed, our breathing becomes shallow. With shallow breathing, we are unable to oxygenate and detoxify our cells and tissues effectively. This can lead to the stagnation of energy. This can cause foggy thinking, furthering our state of stress, which aggravates the breathing cycle. This blocks the flow of vitality—both energetically and physically. This can increase feelings of emotional vulnerability. The lack of detoxification of the brain and body can cause fatigue and lethargy. This can drive us to consume caffeine and processed foods for quick energy, which make the body more toxic, further suppressing vitality, creating a vicious cycle. When vitality decreases, vulnerability to illness increases. The immune system becomes weak and the heart has to work harder in order to oxygenate tissues. The heart has to compensate for the lack of oxygen caused by shallow breathing. This can result in a rapid heart rate, palpitations and high blood pressure. When the brain is not adequately oxygenated, mood is adversely affected causing depression and anxiety.

Just by breathing deeply and consciously, we can purify our bodies and keep our vital flow of life energy from stagnation. In this manner, our breath, a component of our subtle body affects our emotional, mental and physical health.

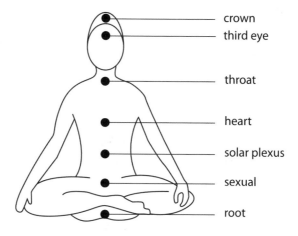

Figure 6: The chakra system

The chakra system

In the East, the anatomy of the body is viewed from both the physical and the energetic levels. A form of medicine that views the anatomy of the Energy body is Chakra Medicine. This is a healing discipline that links concentrated energy wheels in seven areas of the body to nerve and endocrine plexuses (figure 6).

These energy wheels are called "chakras." These are wheels of energy in motion that receive, assimilate and express the energy of

Table 1: The chakras and their corresponding emotions and organs

CHAKRA	LOCATION	EMOTION	ORGAN
1	Base of spine	Feelings of safety, security	Hips, vulva, rectum, sciatic
2	Between pubic bone and belly	Relationship with money, sexual potency, ability to relate to others	Lower back, pelvis, uterus, ovaries, bladder, large intestine, cervix, vagina
3	Solar plexus	Issues of power, fear, self-esteem, trust, self-confidence, self-worth	Abdomen, liver, gall bladder, adrenals, kidneys, pancreas, upper intestine, mid-spine
4	Mid chest	Love, intimacy, judgment, anger, grief	Heart, lungs, breasts, shoulders, esophagus
5	Throat	Self-expression	Throat, thyroid, neck, mouth, teeth, gums, jaw
6	Between the eyebrows	Insight, intuition, knowledge	Brain, pineal gland, eyes, ears, nose
7	Crown of the head	Relationships with spirituality, divinity, humanitarianism, larger perspective	Muscles, skin, nerves, skeleton

the "life force." They are said to contain "bioenergetic" energy, that is, energy that affects the body and is affected by the body. When they are spinning, the chakras are moving bioenergetic energy. When they are stagnant, the bioenergetic energy is blocked at their anatomical level. A sensation of bioenergetic movement would be the feeling of "butterflies in the stomach." This corresponds to the 3rd chakra or the solar plexus chakra in rapid motion. An orgasm is the feeling of the bioenergetic life force flowing through the chakras.

The chakras are an aspect of the subtle body system. Consciousness flows through the chakras, and their movement in turn, affects consciousness. When we become stressed or emotionally stuck, this affects the movement of the chakras that correspond to the emotions we feel. When their energy stagnates, it affects the organs that correspond to them. This stagnation manifests in the Emotional, Mental and then Physical bodies. Specific emotional characteristics that corresponding to the chakras are shown in Table 1.

When our chakras become blocked, we are impacted at many levels and become vulnerable to illnesses. As we bring awareness to the issues that correspond to effected chakras, we can orient ourselves in a healing process that has precision and meaning.

Joan

Joan is a 43-year-old woman who came to see me due to the sudden onset of diabetes and an unexplained increase in body weight. She had been healthy for most of her life, exercised regularly, and enjoyed a diet abundant in whole and minimally processed foods. She did not understand the cause for her diabetes or weight gain and was discouraged because nothing she changed in her lifestyle altered her blood sugar or weight. She followed a diabetic diet without success. She felt "stuck" and mildly depressed due to feelings of hopelessness about her condition.

When I connected the emotional issues of *power, fear and*

self-esteem that corresponded to her third chakra with the pancreas, she began to realize that her issues with blood sugar ran deeper than just the physical level. The pancreas is an organ that corresponds to the third chakra. It is the endocrine organ that secretes insulin that regulates the metabolism of blood sugar. This organ is influenced by the emotional issues that correspond with the third chakra.

Although Joan was living a healthy lifestyle, she had not addressed the issues resulting from her low self-esteem that continued to surface in her life that now manifested with greater vigor in her forties. She had been abused as a child and had lived in fear for most of her life. She was constantly afraid of making a mistake and being punished for it. Her sense of self relied upon how she was treated by others, and she lived in constant fear of being punished, for not being "good enough." This fear was the primary emotion that held her hostage, eroded her self-esteem, and blocked her third chakra. The stagnation she experienced at this level affected her adrenal glands. Her on-going low grade, fight-or-flight response as a result of this fear caused her adrenals to regularly produce stress hormones which led to an increase in her blood sugar. It also impaired the production of insulin by blocking the "flow of vitality" to her pancreas which was not working in a healthy manner. In our work together, I helped her become aware of her constant fear and recommended a Reiki therapist to identify where she felt it in her body in order to release its energy from that area.

Reiki is a form of energy work that can help restore the chakras to healthy flow. It is likened to a massage only without touch. It is a massage of the Energy body. The intention of the Reiki therapist is critical to the efficacy of their work. As the intention to restore healing to the patient is upheld through the session, the technique of Reiki can release the energy of contaminating issues that block the body's energy.

Joan also needed to work through self-esteem issues in psychotherapy. As Reiki released the energy that resulted from fear and caused her low self-esteem, through her work in psychotherapy, she was able to identify the disempowered areas in relationship to herself that she needed to reintegrate and reclaim. It made her therapeutic process more effective in a shorter period of time. Within three months, her blood sugar began to normalize and she began to lose weight. Within six months, her blood sugars were consistently normal and she was twenty pounds lighter. She was well on her way to a healthy future.

Joan's healing was deeper than just the physical reversal of her diabetes. She reclaimed herself from the chronic fear that controlled her behavior through Reiki and psychotherapy. As her third chakra began to heal, her fear was released and her self-esteem was restored. Her 3rd chakra stagnation was healed through the awareness she gained from the expertise and support of her therapists. She learned strategies and tools in psychotherapy that raised her awareness and helped her understand and dismantle her fear. She healed the stagnant third chakra through Reiki. Her life energy began to flow and she became more confident and empowered.

Diabetes had been the catalyst that brought her awareness to her third chakra issues. She courageously worked through these in order to redefine herself. As she worked through her process, her fear no longer contaminated her relationship to her real self. She connected with her intrinsic power and healed the diabetes as an added benefit to the deeper healing that she worked hard to achieve. Her empowered presence could now benefit others in ways she could not have even imagined before her healing process began. The awareness of her subtle body and its need for balance was critical to her core healing.

Working with patients and practitioners from this framework for the past two decades has broadened my perspective of health and illness beyond just the Physical body. It has provided me with insight and awareness to ask questions that identify the causal levels of imbalance. This has assisted me in making referrals to the appropriate practitioners who can then work with patients to restore balance at these levels. When combined with traditional medical tools, this frequently brings the patient's Four Body System into alignment. When alignment and balance are achieved, true healing can be experienced. This also facilitates a level of awareness in the patient to be able to make healthier choices on a daily basis, and broadens their depth of wisdom, assisting them to live more consciously.

Clearly, there is no single solution to health or illness. We are multi-layered organisms who live in energy fields that are constantly changing. We are constantly processing information at many levels. We are influenced by the food we eat, the traumas we bear, the support we receive and the choices we make. Our choices greatly influence our health. If we seek and choose from a place of self-advocacy, we are less likely to get sick. If we choose from complacency or compensations, we are more likely to get sick. We go through life transitions that have significant impacts on our health. The interrelationships between biology, biography, emotions and energy greatly affect our health.

The meridian system of energy

Eastern philosophy is based on the premise that all life occurs within the cycle of nature. Things within this nature are connected and mutually dependent on each other. Nature is one unified system, the Tao with polar and complementary aspects: Yin and Yang. Nature is in constant motion, following cyclic patterns that describe the process of transformation. When the elements of nature are in balance, life is harmonic and flourishes. When the balance of the polar forces is upset, disaster looms.
~Harriet Beinfield and Efrem Korngold

The Chinese coined the term *Qi* to mean basic stuff, or the "stuff that makes things happen," or "stuff in which things happen." It is the life force or life energy that flows through energy channels or meridians in the body in precise patterns that effect health and well-being. If the flow of *Qi* is blocked, life flow stagnates and illness results. In order to restore a state of health, the restoration of the flow of *Qi* within the meridians is necessary.

In order for us to be healthy, the Chinese believe that we must be able to adapt to our environment with a level of harmony that keeps our nature balanced. When this harmony is disrupted, our resources are exhausted and we become sick. They say, "The man is not sick because he has an illness, he has an illness because he is sick."

Just as imbalance in a garden caused by too much heat, water, dryness or lack of sunlight effects the growth of the plants, excess or inadequate *Qi*, excess heat or dampness, inadequate nutrition or poor circulation of *Qi* weakens our health. The doctor is likened to a gardener whose role is to restore the soil to health. As a result, the garden becomes healthy. In the same manner, the doctor's role is to help bring balance to excess heat, moisture or dampness in the body in order for the *Qi* to flow adequately. This is done through acupuncture, herbs, nutritional and lifestyle changes. In order to sustain balance, flow is necessary. This is where the doctor's recommendations create additional impact. Her acupuncture treatments that insert very thin needles at specific points along the meridians can restore the flow of *Qi* and bring well-being back into the system.

Yin and Yang:
As mentioned earlier, two main aspects of our nature are Yin and Yang energies. The Yin and Yang aspects are integral to the balance of the Energy body. The Yang aspect is fast, erratic, light and hot. The Yin aspect is slow, deliberate, cool, dense and persevering. When there is too much Yang, our body suffers from excess heat. Some of the symptoms of too much Yang are hot flashes, night sweats, acid reflux, dry and cracked skin, anxiety and rapid heart rate. Too much Yin is associated with a slow pace, reduced metabolism, cool skin and fatigue.

Our internal organs correspond to Yin energy and our outer skin and muscles correspond to Yang energy. The upper body corresponds to Yang and the lower body, rooted in the earth, corresponds to Yin. Yin provides the substance required to sustain Yang. Without it, the Yang is weakened, and the body is unprotected. Yin and Yang mutually support each other. This is also necessary for sustained health and flow of *Qi*.

Yin energy naturally stagnates during midlife. As the body prepares to enter the second half of life and to slow itself down from the high Yang activity of youth, the body becomes somewhat imbalanced and needs more focused attention to restore and maintain balance. Restoring the flow of Yin and Yang channels, and supporting the Yin channels that are receding and stagnant, are necessary for health and vitality. If a woman ingests foods high in Yang energy such as processed foods, coffee and alcohol, she is more likely to have the typical menopausal symptoms common in the Western hemisphere. It would serve her well to see an acupuncturist, balance her diet, take Chinese herbs (prescribed by a licensed acupuncturist), and replenish her Yin energy for restoration of health and well-being. If she does not make the changes in her lifestyle necessary to maintain the balance of Yin and Yang energies, it may be more difficult for her to truly restore her health.

> Health as defined as the poised balance between Yin-Yang, and sickness is the result of a deficiency or excess, a Yin-Yang disharmony. Survival is based on an organism's capacity to adapt to changing conditions and maintain equilibrium. Yin-Yang harmony is a metaphor for sustaining adaptability and equilibrium.
> ~Harriet Beinfield and Efrem Korngold

Chris

Chris is a 48-year-old woman who had been on natural hormones. According to her blood levels, her hormones were well-balanced, but she continued to suffer from hot flashes, night sweats and insomnia. She had difficulty falling asleep and when she did, she awakened around 3 a.m. with anxiety. She was perplexed with her symptoms and came to me for help.

Chris was working in a stressful job and was tired and depleted at the end of the day. She ate fast food for lunch, washed it down with soda, and drank multiple cups of coffee to maintain her energy. For dinner, she ate a high fat meal followed by a nightcap in order to comfort her anxiety and relax. She craved sugar and found herself snacking on candy and chocolate quite frequently.

From her symptoms, it was clear that Chris was "overheated." She needed help to reduce the excess heat generated from her highly Yang diet, and she needed a series of acupuncture sessions in order to restore flow to her Yin channels which were stagnant and deficient.

After eight sessions of weekly acupuncture and changes in her diet and lifestyle, her symptoms began to heal. She switched to a diet high in Yin energy consisting of whole grains and root vegetables and removed alcohol, processed foods and coffee, all high in Yang energy, from her diet. Within two months she was cured of the symptoms that had initially brought her in to see me. Her symptoms returned if she re-introduced the Yang foods that she had eliminated. Her symptoms did not return if she followed the lifestyle that kept her energy balanced and her *Qi* flowing through her meridian channels.

The Emotional body

I have been particularly interested in the Emotional body as our culture encourages us to deny it and often considers it as pathological. We sometimes think our deep and intense feelings are a sign that we are ill, and we shame people for being "emotional." We often apologize for our feelings of sadness or grief. Our feeling function is our connection to our hearts and our instincts. It tells us what feels right or wrong. We have created a multibillion dollar industry of pharmaceutical medications that suppress our feeling function. Our Emotional body may be the most important body that connects us with what is real. It is the conduit to our souls. If we deny or suppress it, we lose our capacity to heal the Energy body.

The Emotional body is the body that informs us that our Energy body is traumatized, overloaded or imbalanced. It tells us when we are not safe, and it warns us through our instincts if we are in harm's way. If we obey society's rules of closed systems, and deny or suppress our feeling function, we often risk our health and sometimes even our lives. The Feminine Principle can only be accessed through our feeling function. A fully integrated and validated Emotional body expresses the wisdom of the Feminine Principle.

After spending half of our lives denying our Emotional bodies in order to feel accepted by society, we often find ourselves with deeply charged feelings towards issues that we adapted to during the first half of our lives. We start to lose tolerance for pettiness and for certain behaviors we adapted to before this juncture. As our hormones shift, our feeling function rises. Our Emotional bodies become more palpable and more sensitive during this time.

I have observed how a woman's sensations in her body and the sensitivity of her nervous system are profoundly impacted by the fall in progesterone levels. She can sense things in ways she has not been able to since childhood. Perimenopausal women tell me that they feel like a "ball of nerves." They cry during commercials. Their expressed feelings are deeper and more intense than ever before. They have difficulty containing and understanding this new level of feeling function. This frightens many who have been emotionally repressed or who have denied their feelings for half of their lives. They react and respond to issues in ways they never thought they could. They are surprised at their ability to speak their truth. This is a new aspect of character for many women who have held their truth inside and have adapted to the truth of others. They experience a new sense of freedom and empowerment. This is who they really are underneath the compensations and adaptations they have acted from in order to be accepted. They are finally able to feel and experience the beauty of their intrinsic power. They transform into women who can no longer deny their strong feeling function.

The Mental body

If women hold their feelings and their truths inside during midlife, they are much more vulnerable to depression and anxiety. The emotional repression builds internal pressure that "spills over" into the Mental body. It affects the production of serotonin in the brain and nervous system; it causes them to feel restless. This is what sometimes brings women to the psychiatrist's office for healing. Psychiatric medications can palliate the symptoms of depression and anxiety, but they are unable to empower women to express the truth connected to their deep feeling function. In fact, medications do the opposite. It is important for us to understand the *causes* of mental symptoms during menopause and work with the Emotional body to first understand and then process them in order to free this body from repressed and invalidated feelings. One of my patients was appropriately weaned off her antidepressants over a six month period and quit her unfulfilling job after she discontinued them. She said she was unable to adapt to the toxic work environment without the numbing effects of anti-depressants. She is much happier now and her ability to sense dysfunction has reawakened.

I believe many of our mental symptoms have their origins in the Emotional body. They are expressed in the Mental body, as the Emotional body is given no framework or validity in our culture. For as long as we normalize the suppression of our feeling function and hold the perception that denying our feelings is a sign of "strength," the Emotional body will become imbalanced and express symptoms. If we self-medicate in order to reduce these symptoms, we risk becoming vulnerable to addictive patterns, furthering our state of ill mental health.

The field of psychiatry is effective and critical to the treatment of *true* mental illness. When I refer to the inadequacy of psychiatric medications in helping symptoms due to hormonal imbalance, I am not speaking of *true* mental illness. I am referring specifically to the common symptoms of anxiety and depression that often accompany perimenopause and menopause. These symptoms need a framework for understanding, and release and balance. The majority of them are not due to *true* mental illness.

The Physical body

$$E = mc^2$$
~Albert Einstein

Albert Einstein stated that energy and mass are equivalent. It takes linear time for energy to congeal into mass. If the Energy body is imbalanced in specific ways, it will manifest its imbalance in the Physical body with precision.

The traditional medical model views illness only through the lens of the Physical body. Its focus is on the physical repair needed through diagnosis and treatment. Our medical education and cultural framework do not include an evaluation of the *causes* for illness. Causes are considered only at physical levels and are confused with their *manifestation*. Deeper causes are not explored that may be integrally connected to illnesses that manifest in the Physical body. "Disease" is not viewed from the perspective of imbalance. It is viewed from the perspective of biological breakdown. Hence, treatments involve manipulations of only the Physical body through surgery or medications. These may be able to fix the physical symptoms and offer relief, but they do not affect *true* healing. Furthermore, patients begin to rely on medications for symptom management. They are costly and do not heal the causes of illness. If patients are not able to understand these causes, their healing remains incomplete.

Most of our suffering due to illness results from our inability to access the imbalances at deeper levels which *manifest* with precision as symptoms in our physical bodies. When we do not heal the imbalances in the energy and Emotional bodies, they manifest in the Physical body. We cannot *heal* our suffering through physical means alone. This needs deeper levels of healing.

We can liken the Four Body System framework to different expressions of the molecular structure of water, H_2O. It can be expressed in different densities as steam, water or ice. At different densities it is still H_2O. Steam can be likened to the Energy body, water to the Emotional and Mental bodies and ice to the Physical body. If the steam is contaminated, this contamination will be present in the water and ice that it turns into. In the same way, we are a continuum of energy that expresses itself at different densities. An imbalance or "dis-ease" in the Energy body will express itself in the Physical body.

As we expand our perspective of the body to include its emotional and energetic aspects, we will be able to restore health, healing and harmony to our lives at all levels. This expanded perspective of health has the capacity to evoke the seeker in us. Through this new and expanded lens, we can look for areas of imbalance that run deeper than just mental or physical levels that may need core healing. This can bring us a greater level of consciousness and can restore meaning and precision to our process.

It is necessary for women in midlife to advocate for balancing their four bodies for restoration of health and to find practitioners and healers who can help them achieve this. It is also important for traditional physicians to expand their traditional tool box and their diagnostic skill set to include ways of viewing and treating illness that include the Energy, Emotional and Mental bodies in order to *truly* heal and empower patients more effectively. This framework is truly integrative and describes the practice of integrative medicine more completely.

Additional medical training is not necessary in order for physicians to effectively practice integrative medicine. What they actually need is a broader and more comprehensive framework for diagnosis and treatment, one that views illness and health as influenced by a multileveled system in the patient. They must be able to expand their physical framework to include the treatment and balance of all levels that affect health, and recommend appropriate and certified practitioners to assist in the restoration of balance. Physicians who are briefly trained in complementary disciplines and then claim expertise in them undermine the art, skill and expertise of practitioners with extensive training in these disciplines, who practice them as their life's work.

The framework of the Four Body System has the potential to change the face of health care by reducing costly treatments that only address the physical level in an attempt to "fix" illnesses, when their causes arise from deeper levels in the body. This can also deepen the level of care that physicians provide to their patients as they both seek answers to the crucial questions that illness evokes. Both physicians and patients will be enriched by the process of exploration at causal levels. Patients could be active participants in their process and the current fear-based relationships with their physicians could transform into partnerships serving the original and sacred intention of healing and inner growth that has been lost in our current health care system.

In a system where physician burnout is at an all-time high, this expanded paradigm of diagnosis and treatment can offer a much deeper level of fulfillment. This has the potential to open our closed system of medicine and provide a richer perspective towards life. This could facilitate our society to live with an awareness of the importance of restoring balance for the reclamation of health.

6

What Is Love?

Love

What do you call love?
There is a strange definition of it,
infected by the unholy
surface of the mask.
That is not love.
That is—
Living from the shell
without knowledge of
the animal that breaths beneath,
that crawls close to the earth,
and feels warmth and sand, dirt and mud.
Love is that—
becoming that animal
breathing the sacred breath beneath the skin
when it breaks through its shell,
leaving scars and pain, grief and LIFE.
Love is—
a communion
with the mess of it all.
It never closes.
It has sound of the wail released by the mother,
as the baby rips out into the world.
It has the sound of a grief cry
when there is loss.

It brings out laughter and joy—
and all the things that feed
the hungry ghosts and lay them to rest.
Love is not some fillet companionship.
It brings out what is buried
and exposes what is hidden—
the things that betray life.
The love I feel is not a mask;
but a deep cauldron that,
while holding the mess of it all,
offers beauty to life.
It is an opening to the sublime,
a portal to what is Holy.
It can hold everything transforming
and never closes or dies.

To love oneself is the beginning of a life-long romance.
~Oscar Wilde

As we approach midlife, we find ourselves reacting to our loved ones in ways that are unfamiliar and sometimes startling. The deep midlife transformation underway in our psyches causes this. It attempts to connect us with our authentic selves. Our old definitions for what we value and how we relate are called into question to reframe and purify. We find that we need to dive underneath these familiar definitions and connect with their deeper meaning in ways that resonate with our truth, not the one that society has defined for us. Sometimes we find that our truth is contrary to society's definition which creates a tension within us that can feel disheartening and difficult. It is no longer possible for us to deny our truth and live from obedience to social norms if they do not resonate with who we really are. It becomes difficult in midlife for us to allow society to define us.

Susan

Susan is a 45-year-old woman who came to see me after a year of worsening perimenopausal symptoms. She was confused and frightened by her newly felt anger towards tasks she had happily performed for many years, such as picking up after her children and preparing dinner when her husband arrived home from work. She worked from nine to five in customer service for a department store. She was emotionally depleted after dealing with dissatisfied customers. In addition, she felt depleted by the dysfunctional dynamics at work. Her job was unfulfilling and she no longer found meaning in her work. It was merely a means for making a living. After a hard day, she would come home to a mess, which her teenage children did not help her clean, and to a husband who was tired, hungry and expected a cooked dinner and a clean house. She had been tolerant towards this for sixteen years, but started to feel agitation and anger towards the unjust treatment she felt that she had adapted to. She felt she was expected to perform these tasks as her "duty" as a wife and mother, in addition to her full time job. When she made her discontent known to her husband and children, they told her that she needed a "shrink" to fix her because there was something wrong with her. She was acting "crazy" and with "too much" emotion. This discontent was unlike her prior nature and they wanted her to behave in the ways that they had become used to.

Love defined as self-sacrifice

Susan was beyond frustration. Like many of us who have been programmed to obey society's expectations for the sake of "duty" while sacrificing our own needs, we suddenly find ourselves angry with these expectations, sometimes for the first time in midlife. We realize that for many years we undermined our own needs in favor of what was expected from us. We were conditioned to not question these expectations, and were considered "good girls" if we sacrificed our needs in favor of the needs of others. Self-sacrifice was an awarded behavior. It was mistakenly defined for us as "love." We learned to second-guess any inner resistance that we felt towards this unhealthy pattern. We saw women behaving from this definition of "love" everywhere we looked. We were outnumbered when we questioned this behavior as unhealthy. We learned to undermine our questioning. We lost trust in our deepest wisdom, our instinct and intuition.

As children, when we felt the dissonance between our inner wisdom and society's expectations and expressed this conflict to our parents, we were told to stop questioning and adapt to what was expected. We did this in order to be accepted and feel safe. Over time, these became our adapted patterns. We learned to stop questioning. We understood that the virtuous place in loving relationships was the place of self-sacrifice. We learned to give without receiving.

When we continue to give without receiving, we feel the imbalance created by this in our Energy and Emotional bodies. Sometimes it manifests as anger. Since we were conditioned to think that overriding our feelings was a virtue, we ignored our questioning for the sake of duty and obedience. When we feel anger because of this in midlife, we actually are experiencing a normal response to an unhealthy pattern which rises in our feeling function, but we are not able to trust that our anger is a sign of health. We feel there is something wrong with us if we question what seems normal for others. Furthermore, society shames us for questioning. When we suppress our emotions, we do not realize that causes us to adapt to society's closed systems. Its definitions and rules override our feelings as we learned to associate love with self-sacrifice. One often defines the other. This disconnects us from our feeling function. Over time, the emotional pressure caused by this builds within us and as it attempts to release, our midlife journey begins. We are longer able to contain this pressure. We call this rage.

The Emotional body would not suffer in this way if we were taught that giving and receiving are both necessary for healthy love, and that anger is a sign of health. Questioning and examining society's definitions are also signs of health, and trusting the wisdom in our feeling function is a prerequisite for self-respect. The Emotional body can no longer hold the charge resulting from the suppression of our truth and wisdom in midlife. This charge is regarded by many as pathological. This charge is the fury that results from continual disobedience of the real self in favor of society's rule that do not resonant with our truth. This charge is what we are punished for, what we punish ourselves for, and what we need to understand and work with in order to release. Held within this charge is the call for us to be true to ourselves and to honor our needs and redefine the meaning of love. This takes courage. If we don't do this, we become depressed. The Emotional body's imbalance begins to "seep into" the Mental body. This manifests as symptoms that bring many to the physician's office for help.

We are collectively caught in loops that result from our childhood imprinting. We were imprinted with society's definition of love. Through this imprint, we learned how to serve others without question, without boundaries, without balance and without exchange. This is not love in its truest sense, but society's distortion of love that defines love as self-sacrifice and we are conditioned to adapt to this. These become our normalized and familiar patterns.

The self-*lessness* that has contaminated our definition of love is not love. It is over-care. We have confused over-care with love. Over-care is a word that means caring too much for the other. Over-care dis-empowers all who participate. When we over-care for others in relationships, we unconsciously assume that they are unable to care for themselves. We think that they rely on *us* for their care. Unknowingly we dis-empower them. This is the definition of rescue, not love. When we were being imprinted with this pattern and learned to relate in these ways, this felt unhealthy. Since we were taught to distrust our feeling function, we ignored how we felt and continued this pattern of rescue. Any thought of self-care that rustled inside was dismissed as selfish. Self-care is what the Emotional body craves and needs in order to stay balanced and maintain health.

Along with anger, a feeling of "loss of self" results from many years of self-sacrifice. This is a feeling that all women know in their hearts, but are unable to define. What we have given of ourselves to others in "the name of love" compromises our connection to our authentic selves. When our anger and irritation arise, we feel lost and disoriented. This is a new and frightening feeling that creates confusion towards our inability to operate from familiar rules at this juncture. I believe this is the manner in which our soul informs us that we cannot pour ourselves forth "for the sake of love" and expect nothing in return. We cannot live in this way and expect to feel whole. We cannot compromise our integrity and expect our relationships to be healthy. We cannot compromise our sovereignty in an attempt to normalize society's rules. Our souls call to us for course corrections back to our truth.

We are conditioned by society's standards

There is a term used in psychology called operant conditioning. This is a form of psychological learning where individuals modify their behavior due to a stimulus delivered upon the expression of certain behaviors. When a person in a position of authority punishes us with noxious consequences for certain behaviors, we learn to not behave those ways. When they reward us for certain behaviors, we learn to behave in those ways. Some rewards, such as praise and acceptance (by authority) are enough for us to perform the behaviors associated with these rewards. In these situations, the person in the position of authority has power over us. We quickly learn the behaviors that offer rewards and those that offer punishments. We adapt to society in these ways, through operant conditioning.

When we were young, we learned the rules of life from our families. Our families were our small universes that prepared us to function in the world with their patterns of behavior. These patterns were modeled to us by our mothers, fathers, teachers, the media, and our culture at large. They were reinforced through rewards and punishments. Often, the reward was acceptance; the punishment was rejection. Physical and emotional violence are both forms of punishment when they are associated with specific behaviors. We quickly learned to avoid punishment. Since we all craved connection, we learned to define "right" and "wrong" behaviors in this manner. We became imprinted and programmed by our family's definitions through operant conditioning.

Many of us watched our mothers sacrifice themselves and over-care for others. We also witnessed them becoming depressed and anxious in midlife. We heard them rationalizing their over-care and normalizing it with their friends, other midlife women. They were not able to see their symptoms as a sign that they needed reframing and renewal. They did not have a relative position for health.

Since we were raised this way, we struggle with the ominous feeling that we will end up like our mothers. We need to understand the meaning of their symptoms and their struggle between the needs of their real selves and the demands of society. They did not have a vocabulary or a framework to define their needs and feelings in ways that we do. We need to use our vocabulary and redefine ourselves at this juncture in midlife. We need to consider self-care as a major priority. We need to trust our feeling function and the wisdom it holds. We need to redefine health. A deeper challenge for many women is the belief that their needs are not important. They often confuse this as a belief that *they* are not important. This injunction leads us to believe that our needs are secondary to the needs of others—that our purpose in life is to serve others. This is the furthest from our soul's truth.

This truth awakens during midlife and marks our journey back to ourselves. For many women, this journey is marked by breast cancer. Women who fail to nurture themselves are at risk for diseases of their breasts. Many of my patients who developed breast cancer in midlife felt that their cancer was a symptom of their depleted Energy bodies and a call from their Emotional bodies for self-nourishment. They feel that this deeper cause of their cancer resulted from a lifetime of selfless service to others. It was a wakeup call for them to look at the imbalances in their Energy bodies that were depleted from sacrificing their boundaries along with a lack of self-care. This was their body's way of awakening them to deeper imbalances which manifested symbolically. As they explored these levels of cause, they were able to reclaim their worth and validate their needs. For some, it involved the experience of transforming these patterns through illness in order to reconnect to self, to come home to self, and to honor the needs of self. In the U.S., one in seven women will be diagnosed with breast cancer every year. We must address these energetic causes by learning how to balance giving with receiving. This can be a life-saving pattern for all of us.

What does this have to do with love?

This has everything to do with love. The basic fabric of love is encoded in our hearts. We know this innately. But, we are conditioned to forget this. We live from unhealthy definitions of love normalized by society. We become unhealthy ourselves when we behave in these ways. If we behave from society's definitions of love we lose our personal boundaries. We lose contact with our limits—where we end and another begins. Women tell me that they are unable to stop this cycle.

Women in our culture are not taught how to be feminine except in relationship to men. Women allow men to define this for them. This definition is an extension of society's distorted definition of the feminine which is superficial and incomplete. The relationships women have with themselves are heavily influenced by cultural definitions, which leave them feeling empty and disconnected. This is an epidemic in our society. This wounds women and makes them vulnerable to abuse where others define and control their behavior. When women are disconnected from what is real for them, they are also disconnected from their intrinsic power and abdicate it to others. They are unable to live from their truth in this dynamic.

In extreme cases, we stay in abusive marriages as a result of our conditioning. We continue to serve in unhealthy jobs and tolerate disrespect for the sake of "love for our families." As a woman who lived from these definitions, I realized in retrospect that all the ways in which I defined myself through them made me vulnerable to abuse. My instinct for boundaries was wounded and I second-guessed my needs and placed the needs of others at the forefront. I was unknowingly betraying my needs like many women do. My midlife process forced me to awaken to these unhealthy patterns and to dismantle them in order to redefine who I needed to become.

Love is a feeling

In the English language, there is only one word for love. In Inuit, there are 23 words for love. In the East, there are close to 50 words for love. In countries where English is the primary spoken language, the definition of love is vulnerable to distortion. Here, the same word for love defines the love for one's child, spouse, pet, parents, friends, material goods, weather, home or job. In the East, the description of different kinds of love is qualified with sensory undertones and poetic expressions. There are different meanings and inflections when love is described. The different forms of love evoke different feelings within. In the Western hemisphere, since feeling function is not valued, our descriptions of love have become vulnerable to distortion and contamination. With our wounded feeling function, we have become conditioned to use this word as society defines it for us.

The Western definition of love does not embody feeling. The qualities of truth and integrity are not seen as integral components of its current definition. These are core qualities that reside in the heart alongside love. Love is the energy that emanates from the heart. Fierce love is fearless and resilient. It is active, not passive. It requires behaving in ways that strengthen health and healing within both self and in others. Tough love, like fierce love, behaves in ways that transcend the fear of conflict. It is committed to doing what is best for others despite their displeasure when it is expressed. It is able to hold a standard for others, set from a place of integrity. It has faith in the power of truth. It evokes patience and is able to endure rejection for the sake of integrity. This kind of love is no stranger to parents of teenagers. Our difficult journeys with them teach us about this kind of love. This is a love we all deserve. It arises from a deep place of feeling and is not satisfied with any level of compromise. It is the kind of love that awakens in most women in midlife in relationship to themselves. It is worth exploring and is worthy of reintegrating into the fabric of our being. It has within it the power to restore self-respect and self-esteem. It teaches us to honor our feelings and to not compromise our integrity or truth for anyone. It can even heal us from abuse.

What love is not

> No person is your friend who demands your silence,
> or denies your right to grow.
> ~Alice Walker

We need to ask ourselves where our integrity is when we sacrifice ourselves for society's rules for acceptance. If we are expected to compromise, disrespect, shame, undermine and deplete ourselves or are expected to subdue our wisdom or our feeling function, we are not behaving from self-love. If duty expects this of us, then we must reevaluate whether this is healthy or not. Love and health are synonyms. We must integrate its healthy definition into our behaviors.

In my former relationship, I was asked if I would rather be "right or alone" when I spoke my truth strongly. Love would have held a space for my truth to be received and heard. I was threatened with rejection and abandonment when I spoke my truth. I was conditioned very quickly to keep my mouth shut to serve the definition of love that I was expected to embody. My imprinted self did not argue with this. This was familiar. It is confusing to know how to behave when we are conditioned.

Many women who are imprinted with distorted definitions from society define love as "compliance to the system" within which they reside, whether at home or at work. They are taught through their conditioning to not question the lack of health in these systems. These systems are closed systems. In closed systems, its unhealthy members in positions of authority define love in unhealthy ways, confusing the intrinsic love of truth and integrity, with duty and obedience. They demand secrecy for the sake of "love" from the systems members, and expect them to adapt to the system's rules. These unhealthy members are the ones who define love as compliance to the system. This is not love. This is manipulation. Unless we understand this, we stay vulnerable to losing contact with our real selves in favor of these ways of thinking and behaving. After behaving this way for years, we may consider this as "normal." Midlife changes all of this. Our psyches and souls speak to us through our feeling function and begin to dismantle these false definitions. Since connecting with others is like oxygen for many, the terror of losing connection through this act of redefinition can be daunting.

We have to remember the truth of who we are and our faith must reside in this. Our fear of separation from others is worth the joy of reconnecting with our real selves. If people leave our lives as we identify with what is real, then we must question the health of these relationships. As we leave them behind, our commitment to our own health will draw in relationships that we resonate with from authenticity and meaning. We have to remember this. When we enable relationships that normalize the rules of closed systems, we become a part of the problem, not the solution. Redefining ourselves involves dismantling our conditioned adaptations. If we do not do this consciously, the pressure that has built within us from living without connection to our truth will arise from our Energy and Emotional bodies in the form of a "crisis." This is guaranteed in midlife. Our Energy and Emotional bodies call for both balance and healing from adaptations that do not resonate with our truth. Our soul calls us to live from our true purpose. Without this process of reframing and reclaiming, we are unable to live authentically. Indigenous people consider this process a form of soul retrieval. Without engaging this process, we endanger the remainder of our lives with feelings of emptiness and we risk adversely affecting the lives of those we love with our unmet needs.

Sentimentality confused as love

Carl Jung defined sentimentality as a "superstructure covering brutality." I believe he was saying that covering our authentic selves by distorted definitions removes our connection to feeling. This puts us at risk for "brutal" behavior. This can result when we compromise our feeling function through adaptions to society's rules that lead our disconnection to our real self. Authentic feeling from the Emotional body is not present in sentimentality. It is the theoretical understanding of the word "love" without the depth of feeling as described earlier. Sentimentality is behaved through the distorted definitions of love without truth and integrity which is an integral part of true love.

Sentimentality risks nothing. It does not arise from the heart like love does. Love in its purest form takes risks. Love makes us vulnerable. By nature, love is messy. We risk a broken heart when we love deeply. But in order for us to find meaning and fulfillment in relationships, love must flow from the heart. Sentimentality does not share this quality. Sentimentality does not risk true feeling.

Love is a verb. It is behaved in our relationships with others. Sentimentality is a noun. It is not behaved in relationships with others.

For example, parents who tell their children that they love them, but fail to offer them time and presence are sentimental. A partner, who verbally expresses love, but is unwilling to offer support through difficult times is operating from sentimentality, not love.

Sentimentality is not connected to the Emotional body or feeling function. By nature, it is cool and theoretical. It arises from the mind, not the heart. It lacks passion and emotion. It is not authentic, nor is it connected to the real self. It is an extension of the adapted self. In some families, sentimentality is mistaken for love. When people are imprinted with sentimentality rather than love, they are unable to offer authentic love in relationships. Their relationships remain superficial. When they are in the presence of authentic love, they become frightened. It feels unfamiliar and risky. They avoid it and as a result they miss the experience of depth and meaning in relationships.

Most people who carry this imprinted pattern suffer from depression, as their hearts are not engaged in relationships in a real way. They substitute what is sentimental for what is real and feel empty. If they awaken to this later in life, their journey to loving authentically can be difficult. They have to be willing to take risks in order to experience real love in relationships. If they have the courage to dismantle this imprinted pattern, they can offer themselves the experience of depth and meaning. It is our task in midlife to replace what is sentimental with what is real. It is the only meaningful way in which we can spend the second half of our lives.

Agitation as a sign of health

All around the world, women in midlife are reconsidering the definitions of love and power. Like Susan, they feel agitated when they are manipulated into conforming to and performing within closed systems, where women are expected to serve everyone's needs but their own, through over-care and rescue. Their agitation is a sign of health. It is a sign of being part of a closed system whose rules cause disconnection from the real self. These rules are not based on giving and receiving. They expect self-sacrifice. Women need to pay deep attention to their needs, dismantle their over-caring behaviors and hold a standard of self-responsibility for themselves and others. They must first fill themselves up, and then overflow onto others.

Reclaiming our health

Many women feel that they are being selfish while transforming the familiar dynamic of self-sacrifice into self-nurturing. If depletion is the energetic cause for a disease as severe as breast cancer, we need to take responsibility for healing our energetic imbalances through self-care. We need to incorporate this as a core value into our society.

Our society has a responsibility to support us as we reclaim our health. Our society, being a dysfunctional, closed system, will want to impose its old rules of domination upon us in order to maintain status quo, but without our cooperation it will have to transform into an open system. We must change our behaviors from conditioned ones that make us sick, to ones that honor our real selves and keep us healthy. When we enable society's dysfunctions that are based in fear, we unknowingly collude against ourselves.

A woman's voice and will are the strongest powers on our planet. We must find our voices and assert them on behalf of self-care and health. If we refuse to do this, we will continue to lead our daughters and sons like the Pied Piper, into a river of dysfunction, where love is distorted as self-sacrifice and manifests in symptoms that risk our health. We must transform the sentimental relationships that we may have with ourselves into ones that support self-love through healthy behaviors.

What is healthy love?

Love and health are interdependent. We must dismantle the distorted definitions of love and integrate its healthy meaning into our personal and collective psyches.

Renee

Renee is a 43-year-old woman who came to see me for her symptoms of severe anxiety that began when she discovered that her husband was having an affair. The day after she found out about this, he told her that if she truly loved him she would be happy on his behalf for having found someone he could relate to better than her. This shocked her into examining his definition of love, one that did not resonate with hers. She came to see me to discuss her inner struggle with this, and to validate her definition of love that she felt her husband had violated. This inner struggle was causing her anxiety and insomnia. She felt that his version of love lacked integrity and he was asking her to compromise her version to normalize his betrayal of their marital commitment. She was outraged.

His family, whom she had considered as hers, turned a blind eye to his behavior and asked her to capitulate, to "suck it up," and to "get over" her anger towards him. They even asked her to forgive him. She was unable to forgive his behavior despite their expectations of her. She felt he needed to *earn* her forgiveness by realizing what he had done through true remorse. She wanted him to *feel* this in his heart. If she forgave him without this, she would be colluding with him against herself. She would be enabling his sentimental behavior towards her that normalized betrayal. She would be endangering her integrity and self-respect by "forgiving" his disrespect of their marriage. Her feeling function would not be in alignment with the forgiveness that his family expected. The expectations from his family were a result of sentimentality, not true love. If she "forgave" him for their sake, she would be operating from a place that was not real for her. She realized that his love towards her was sentimental, imprinted and reinforced by the closed system of his family. She was only willing to forgive him if he transformed his sentimentality into real love through remorse, and changed his behavior towards her to one of honor and respect. He never did.

As her feelings were validated, Renee was able to gain comfort from the integrity of her values. She was able to heal her anxiety caused by the inner struggle between her real self and injunctions from others.

Inner resistance

The expectation to compromise integrity for "love" will evoke inner feelings of resistance. If we override these feelings out of obedience to society's expectations, we risk second-guessing our inner wisdom and betraying ourselves. Self-betrayal always manifests in the Emotional and Mental bodies as anxiety or depression. The boundaries mentioned earlier that are necessary for relationships to be healthy sometimes become known to us through our feelings of inner-resistance. These boundaries must be honored. Many women are unable to define their feelings of resistance as healthy boundaries. They have been taught to doubt them. They need to learn to honor them.

Effective therapists can help women walk through this journey back to themselves. Therapists can uncover the causes of depression or anxiety and trace them back to the flawed definitions that women have been living from. They can teach women to honor their inner resistance and to reframe it as a sign of intrinsic health;

a signal from their inner wisdom which warns them of danger to their Emotional and Energy bodies if this feeling is ignored.

Self-talk in most women takes the form of self-criticism or self-doubt. If women pause to listen to these inner-voices, they can erode their healthy relationships to themselves and damage their self-worth. Our imprinting in addition to injunctions from society, take residence in us as our self-talk. This is intimately connected with our feeling function. Most feelings that arise from this critical self-talk do not bring us joy. They cause depression and anxiety and drive us to self-medicate with food, alcohol or shopping. When these distractions do not work, we may take prescribed medications to suppress our feelings. These further disconnect us from our feeling function. True healing requires uncovering the roots of our unhappiness. It requires us to reconnect with ourselves and realign with our truth. In doing this, we can reclaim our happiness and joy.

Love is not rescue

Love does not manipulate others into obedience. This is the definition of manipulation, not love. When one attempts to manipulate and control others in the "name of love," they are operating from the patriarchal construct of domination. This is one of the rules present in closed systems. Since we often mistake rescue for love, we need to be cautious about any hooks that can engage our rescuer. One of these hooks is pity. Women often confuse pity with empathy. They misunderstand empathy to be a sign of love. If pity is being evoked within us, we are on treacherous ground. We are vulnerable to falling into the trap of rescue and mistaking this for love. We unknowingly dominate others through our rescue of them. This act covertly gives us power over them as we do not feel that they can find solutions without us. We believe we can rescue them from their plight. They become dependent on *our* efforts. This is the definition of codependency, not love. Pity hooks many women into codependent relationships.

When they begin their recovery process, women realize in hindsight, that it was pity for the other that hooked them into codependency. They must reclaim themselves from the disempowerment they suffered as a result of this. They mistook pity for empathy. They mistook rescue for love. Pity will evoke feelings of obligation towards others. When we feel obligated to help others in this way, we are in danger of depleting our Energy bodies. Society has conditioned us to confuse this dynamic with love.

Many women who are imprinted with this definition and conditioned by it find themselves in relationships with deeply wounded people. They feel a sense of personal power and purpose as they set out to "heal" the other with their unconditional "love." Many abusive marriages operate from this dynamic. Rescue through over-care will often lead to feelings of entitlement from the other and feelings of resentment if the over-care is withdrawn. This resentment can lead to emotional and physical abuse. Women who are in recovery from domestic violence often see how difficult it was for them to separate themselves from the dysfunctional definitions of love that they behaved from in their unhealthy marriages. Their recovery often involves the redefinition of healthy love and the behaviors that demonstrate it. When they dismantle their rescuer, they are able to restore self-responsibility. This connects them with their intrinsic power. It also helps others become self-responsible in relationship to them.

We need to understand that we are all responsible for our own journeys towards wholeness and health. We are also responsible for our happiness. We must remember this as a basic truth. Our conditioning is in contrast to this. This truth is integral for a healthy life. Another person's happiness is not our responsibility. It is *theirs*. Our love can hold space for others to heal *themselves*. But, for as long as we behave from our rescuer, we engage in over-care, and we risk depletion. The best and the most honorable gift we can offer others is our support and belief in their ability to heal themselves. Their commitment to their journey towards health is honorable and worthy of our support. Their lack of willingness to grow and be self-responsible is a warning for us to not enable them. It will evoke resistance within us. We must behave in accordance with the wisdom of this resistance and honor our boundaries. This is healthy love redefined from an intrinsic place. Love that evokes empowerment is healthy. Love that evokes dependency is not.

Resistance to the closed system is a sign of self-love

A gift of the midlife process is the internal resistance that we feel towards what is not healthy for us. We need to discern our true needs from those we compromise for the sake of duty. The process of learning this can become a spiritual practice. This takes daily awareness. Our disconnected feeling function often begins to awaken when our hormones begin to fall, and the charge buried in the Emotional body rises as internal resistance towards expectations that weigh us down. We need to learn the language of our feeling function. The rules of society have no regard for our *real* needs and in order to redefine ourselves, we must remember the wisdom of our feelings. Once a woman awakens to her internal resistance towards unhealthy patterns, she can never fall asleep again. If she tries, she risks feeling the tension in her Emotional body between her feeling function and the expectations from the closed systems around her.

This tension will aggravate her menopausal symptoms and she may experience an increase in hot flashes, night sweats, insomnia, anxiety or even fatigue. If she does not listen to her feelings, they can also manifest in symbolic ways sometimes through her heart and her breasts. Breasts are symbolic of nurturing and nourishment. The heart where truth, love and integrity reside cannot remain energetically imbalanced for long. It will eventually manifest an illness. Fifty percent of us will suffer heart attacks if we continue to behave from society's definitions and neglect our needs for self-care. We need to attend to the deep needs in our hearts. Purifying our definition of love is one of the ways in which we can begin to heal.

We need to work at the level of the Energy body and redefine ourselves through our deep feelings and dismantle any fears that contaminate our behaviors. We must do this because this is the only way we can transform our culture into one that is feminine-honoring and heart-centered. If we do not behave from a place of self-love, we cannot change the ways in which others treat us. Their treatment is always a reflection of our relationship to ourselves.

The integrity of healthy love

True love takes courage. The root word for courage is "coer," which in Latin means "the heart." Courage resides alongside love within the heart. It enables us to live from integrity despite our fear of rejection. When we are reconfiguring and reframing our systems, we often feel fearful. This is a normal part of transformation. It is important for us to grow our courage greater than our fears and do whatever it takes in order to reframe our lives.

Once our fear passes, our connection to our authentic self will offer us comfort during times when we may feel alone. This is a stage in the journey back to ourselves. A part of this journey is often spent alone. This is a time when we grow inner-eyes. Our instincts begin to heal and we recover our senses and our ability to see reality underneath the illusions around us. We begin to sense what is healthy and what is not. We develop discernment. From this stage forward, we are no longer vulnerable to illusions and will only settle for what feels real. This process can help us to feel safe in our skins and heal our fear of being alone in the world. Through it, we can learn to befriend our real selves.

The danger of familiarity

Too often, we unconsciously recreate dynamics in our adult relationships that we learned from our families of origin. Since most of us do not have a relative position from which to choose, we recreate these dynamics out of familiarity. Many times a feeling of "comfort" with the other may be a wound-based feeling that is familiar. It feels like fusion. Wound-based fusion is often mistaken for resonance. Wound-based relationships are common in our society. They lead to dysfunctional dynamics and codependency. They often fail, as they do not serve the real self. If a relationship like this endures in a marriage, the children raised in this family will be imprinted with a distorted definition of love that is wound-based. They will choose partners from the dynamics they were raised in. Wound-based relationships do not support wholeness or health. People in these relationships must become self-responsible in order to heal. They must do their hard work of recovery. We can never expect the other in a relationship to "complete us" as our society mistakenly tells us they can.

Adults who redefine themselves as separate from their imprinting are adults who have individuated. Seeking and living from one's individuality—separate from the familial imprint—is a difficult and necessary process. This individuation is always difficult because when one attempts to separate from imprinted behaviors, one may feel as though one is betraying one's family of origin. One may feel guilt and shame while doing this. Our souls require us to individuate in midlife in order for us to authentically serve our life's purpose. People who find ways to relate to their families of origin from their individuated selves can stand in their truth and are no longer vulnerable to manipulation by shame or guilt. They learn to relate to their families from a place of sovereignty and from terms based on their truth, the terms that their souls have defined to reclaim their health. Often relationships with their families become more meaningful when they engage with them from their individuated selves.

Love as self-care

Self-love needs to be behaved through acts of self-care. I have observed four ways women can do this to reclaim themselves:

1. Make a commitment to speaking one's truth

2. Make daily exercise a priority

3. Make a commitment to self-nourishment by eating organic and whole foods

4. Invest in a personal growth process that restores balance of the Four Body System

Many women complain that they do not feel worthy enough to spend money on themselves. Some, who are financially dependent on their partners, feel they are undeserving of this expense. They do not want to "rock the boat" in their relationships by caring for themselves. They feel they will be perceived as selfish. Similar comments are not uncommon even from women who support their families! Ultimately, this is an issue of self-worth. Self-worth determines the extent to which we are able to love ourselves. Most women have been shamed into lowering their worth and they view themselves through that lens. When they attempt to elevate their worth in order to heal, they may feel shame. They must reframe the lens of low self-worth that they see themselves through in order to truly heal. They will find this lens to be contaminated by their imprinting and conditioning. Sometimes acts of self-love can release low self-worth contaminations to the surface so women can become conscious of them. Women need to have the courage to do this difficult work. It takes endurance and patience to recalibrate self-worth, but this is necessary in order for us to be able to love from a place of health and authenticity.

Illness forces self-love

Sometimes when faced with a life threatening illness, our priorities shift towards self-care to an extreme. Why should it take a threat from the body to cause us to pay attention to our physical, emotional and energetic needs? Many women find the courage to leave abusive marriages and dysfunctional jobs when diagnosed with life threatening illnesses. They can then reframe their lives and redefine their relationships to themselves and others. The possibility of death has the ability to bring unprocessed "baggage" to the surface for transformation. These women realize that in the end what matters most is how deeply they loved, and the level of integrity they lived from. They feel more at peace if their love was healthy.

A life of distorted love is a life disconnected from what is authentic and real. The greatest gift midlife women can offer themselves and others is healthy love that is real. It is fearless, courageous, and uncompromising. This kind of love is what one leaves as one's legacy. Being in the presence of one who has mastered this can change and transform another into a higher version of themselves. This kind of love is what is necessary and important to heal our hurting world.

This kind of love can only be achieved when we give ourselves permission to speak our truth. We live with the misunderstanding that our truth must be accepted by others. We live from the fear of being rejected and may hold our truth inside and live from a place we are told is "noble" and "honorable." We betray ourselves by doing this and are called to transform this in midlife. Love is able to hold space for our truth. It is necessary for us to speak it. We must express it in order for us to know ourselves and be truly known by others.

Modeling healthy love

As we redefine love towards ourselves, we can model this relationship for others. We have become desensitized as a culture. We spend hours in front of the television living vicariously through its definitions and interpretations of life. We become desensitized to the violence we watch. It causes us to go numb. This wounds our feeling function. Love is not possible without feeling. If we become desensitized to world tragedy and the suffering of others, we become sentimental. This wounds our feeling function which can become like a hungry ghost in its attempt to fill itself through overcompensation by overconsumption. These behaviors deplete us and the earth's resources. We can only be fulfilled through self-love and self-care.

Many women define themselves through the eyes of another. We need to awaken through *our* inner-eyes rather than through those of people around us. It is harder to do this when we are young, as our inner selves are not yet defined. We relied on our parents to define this for us and looked up to them as role models of love. If our parents modeled a distorted or unhealthy system to us, we practiced it in our relationships until it caused us enough pain to awaken to the change that was needed for health. As we redefine ourselves in midlife, we are able to see ourselves more clearly from a real place. From this place, we can individuate.

Our sons and daughters are always watching us. We are mentoring them even when we are unaware. If we raised them with our learned distortions and then transform into our real selves in midlife, we can find solace in knowing that we can offer them a new relative position for health. It will offer them the ability to choose to live from behaviors we model from our new and individuated selves versus the selves that imprinted them with distorted definitions from society.

In my own recovery process, I was able to see how I was conditioned to doubt and second-guess myself. I was not able to connect to myself authentically, and I unknowingly enabled the environment where the Feminine Principle was violated and then betrayed. I awakened to my responsibility for enabling a system where a distorted definition of love was expected. I adapted to this out of fear. Now, I have the capacity to heal myself and my children by reclaiming what is true for me and behaving from this truth. This is the power of self-love. When it is behaved and integrated into our lives, it radiates through our presence. When others are in our presence, they are also able to connect to their authenticity.

When we intrinsically connect to our real selves, our self-worth and self-esteem rises and self-care becomes a priority. This is a curious process that I have keenly observed in my patients. The ones who are able to create this connection to their real selves are able to advocate for themselves through self-care. They do not hesitate to invest in it as they feel they are worth the investment. Self-advocacy arises from self-love. Without self-love one is unable to make a true commitment to health or wholeness as others are valued more than the needs of self. If you find yourself sacrificing self-care for others or making excuses to not invest time or money in self-care, you may need to evaluate your relationship to yourself and your definition of love.

In midlife it becomes easier to reclaim and redefine this as our lack of balance manifests in the form of symptoms. In this way, the wisdom in a woman's body forces her to seek the care she needs in order for her to heal. Most of the care requires the nourishment and balance of The Four Body System. Paradoxically through symptoms, her body attempts to bring a woman into connection with her authentic self.

As midlife women, we owe this to ourselves, each other and especially to our children. When we redefine ourselves in these ways, our systems will begin to value health and empowerment. Through our healing, our families and communities will also heal.

Love and soul

Midlife calls us to connect with our souls. This medial place speaks the language of love that is inseparable from truth and integrity. It is very different than the language of society with its distortions. The soul is uncompromising in midlife and does not rest until we live from it. It becomes our constant guide and does not part ways from us until our deaths.

We need to learn the language of our souls. This language resonates with universal principles of balance and harmony. Our connection to our real selves facilitates behaviors that can fulfill these expectations.

Our souls call us to live in the following ways:

1. To speak our truth and behave from it in our lives
2. To serve our authentic selves by listening to our feeling function
3. To live without compromising integrity
4. To live from truth and honesty in all walks of life
5. To advocate for ourselves through acts of self-care
6. To invest in individuation to dismantle our conditioning
7. To reframe and honor the feelings of resistance as signals of healthy boundaries
8. To love self and others from a place of health and self-respect without compromise
9. To allow others to be self-responsible and not enable them through rescue
10. To listen to our instinct when it warns us of danger to our Energy and Emotional bodies

If you ever feel as though you need to defend yourself or your truth in the presence of another, you are most likely participating in a closed system. It is important for us to trust that our individuation process will transform us for the better. This takes time and requires courage. We need to support each other through this to stay on the path of becoming real in order to fully access our intrinsic power.

Susan revisited

In Susan's journey to self-love, she recognized how she was committing acts of self-betrayal through compromising her truth. She realized how through her obedience of society's definitions of her *duty* as a wife and mother she enabled her family's lack of self-responsibility. She was suffering from depletion and resentment. As fearful as she was to assert her truth to them, she began to express her feelings with the help of support and with the tools she learned in psychotherapy. Her family at first resented this, but soon they began to respect her and follow through with self-responsible behavior. They began to share chores around the house and even helped her prepare dinner. Her husband realized the importance of her need for self-care when she began to behave in ways that demonstrated respect towards herself.

Susan was empowered enough to behave from this dynamic at work. This transformed the treatment she received from her co-workers. She reconfigured the dynamics of all of her relationships and released the ones that did not honor her. She had used her depression as a signal and a catalyst to uncover the dysfunctional relationship that she had with herself. This restored balance in her Energy, Emotional, and Mental bodies, in addition to healing her self-worth. Her depression lifted and she began to live from joy. She began to see her depression as a blessing and gift that helped her grow in ways she never could have before. As an added benefit, I believe she significantly reduced her risk of breast cancer and heart disease.

Redefining love and integrating its healthy definition into our lives is a powerful way for us to transform our communities and our closed systems. We have more intrinsic power than we may think or believe we have. As we commit ourselves to the journey to becoming real, we can make a profound difference in restoring health and wholeness in our wounded world.

7

What Is Power?

My Gift to You
(for my children)

I offer you a gift,
from one who was shaken from terrible suffering.
I am becoming whole.
I have walked through the desert
on my knees for a thousand miles repenting.
I am done with that.
If I am not 'good enough' then so be it.
I offer you the gift of my humanness
and my awakening to
not having always lived from my real self.
I now stand in my Truth.
It is my shield that will keep you safe.
It was violated, betrayed,
and turned to rubble.
I rebuild this shield with my hands, my heart,
my truth and my power.
I reclaim myself in all the places that were shattered.
You help me with your wild rebellion and rage—
medicine for my alchemy.
I offer you this shield.
It will be your fortress and protection.
It will heal the tear.
It will bring you home.

Change is frightening, but where there is fear, there is power.
If we learn to feel our fear without letting it stop us,
fear can become our ally, a sign to tell us that
something we have encountered can be transformed.

~Maureen Murdock

Menopause as an initiation into our intrinsic power

"What is power?" This is an important question in midlife. Most of us feel disempowered by the time we arrive at this stage in life. Women come to see me feeling battered by life. They feel as though they have no voice to express their needs. One woman told me that she wanted to scream without stopping. She said she felt could scream for the rest of her life and it would still not be enough to heal her. She had never connected with her intrinsic power until her hormones began to change. Then she began to feel it. It felt like a pressure inside of her, like a "charge" that had been building due to years of self-denial in obedience to social rules. She said it felt like raw energy. It was her feminine power which had never been given a voice or an outlet. She had never lived from it. She had been busy living a life that was not real for her. Her way of life had been defined by others. She had not awakened to this until her changing biology began to release it into her Energy and Emotional bodies.

Nan

Nan is a 42-year-old woman who was 100 pounds overweight and came to me in hopes of healing her depression and anxiety. She was chronically tired and lived with a feeling of emptiness over the past few years. She had been drinking a glass of wine every night to relax, and when she drank she lost contact with her sensation of fullness. This disconnected her from feeling her limits. She was unaware of the large volumes of food she consumed daily. This behavior had become a pattern over the past year. Her periods were heavy, her libido was low and she hadn't looked at her body in the mirror in eight months. She began to weep in the exam room. "I don't know whose body this is," she said, "I have never been this heavy or felt this awful. It must be my hormones. I think I need a hysterectomy. I just want to stop bleeding and become my old self again. I want my old body back."

She is not unlike many women in their forties when hormonal shifts begin and their deeper bodies awaken to the imbalance within that manifests in mental and physical symptoms. Nan was also going through an identity crisis as her last child was leaving home for college, and her sense of self that was identified with being a mother and a homemaker was threatened. With her children gone, she didn't know who she was. She had been so busy mothering them that she had never stopped to feel her own desires or needs. She did not know who she was apart from being a mother and a wife. She did not know how to begin to explore these issues.

This is a common experience for women in midlife around the world. Not only does their biological identity change, but the roles through which they have defined themselves do as well. They arrive at the "medial place" where Jungians would say women can no longer live from what the world expects of them. They need to live from what their souls expect of them. Like Nan, many women do not even ask these crucial questions. Like Nan, they do not even know how to ask them.

For Nan, the question itself will be a journey through the second half of her life; and no, she will not get her old self back. It was busy serving the world, and did a good job at that. Now the rules of life have changed in this medial place. Even if she found another identity defined for her by the world, it would not fulfill her. She needed to move her focus inward, through framework and strategy so that her midlife journey could become an adventure of self-discovery and restore a sense of connection with herself.

Years ago, I gave a presentation to a large group of midlife executives. I asked them who they were without their families, their jobs, their status, and their homes. Most of the women could not answer the question. They were so identified with the roles that had defined them that they did not know who they were without these roles. They were vulnerable to feeling the emptiness that often marks the midlife gateway. Sometimes this gateway is marked by a crisis. Carried within this "crisis" is hidden its higher purpose—the potential for uncovering who they really are, underneath their assigned and defined roles. This can facilitate the connection to their real selves and their intrinsic power.

Intrinsic power

Intrinsic power is power held within one's truth that differs greatly from the "power principle." In most of our world, power is synonymous with domination. Having power over another gives one the feeling of being powerful. Power over another is the "power principle" at work. This is extrinsic power. In this dynamic, the dominator in the relationship holds power through an externally identified status which may be economic or authoritative. In this case, *fear* is the emotion that regulates the balance of power. This is the kind of power that defines closed systems.

Intrinsic power is inner power. It is felt intrinsically within the fabric of our being when we are in relationships that honor our truth and sovereignty. It does not rely on externally defined roles or those assigned by closed systems. Intrinsic power does not dominate. It is not based in fear and does not evoke fear. This power arises from truth and integrity. Nelson Mandela is an example of a leader with intrinsic power. Although he spent most of his adult life in jail being dominated by the patriarchal system through the "power principle," he never lost connection with his truth or integrity. Gandhi had the same kind of intrinsic power, which he demonstrated throughout his life. His intrinsic power led India into freedom from domination by the British Empire.

Intrinsic power arises from one's connection to the authentic or real self that is *behaved* in one's life. It is not fear-based. It is truth-based and it is connected to one's inner truth and integrity that transcends the fear of rejection. It evokes courage, commitment, endurance, and fearlessness. When one lives from this place, one lives from fierceness. Intrinsic power often threatens the "power principle," as it cannot be dominated.

Women and power

Women are intrinsically powerful. They organically go through a "death and rebirth" cycle every month with menses. This gives them the power to create life. They are able to raise children, build careers, provide nurturing, endure suffering, and can still love fiercely. If they are connected to it, their power can be felt in their presence. A woman's power is the silent power behind the success of their partners and children. Throughout history, they have been the ones that have midwifed birth and death. Their power is intrinsic.

We are imprinted to disconnect from our intrinsic power in closed systems when we are young. All parents imprint their children with their adapted patterns resulting from their own imprinting and conditioning. As children, often when our intrinsic power surfaced in the form of truth telling, we were silenced. If our truth was accompanied by strong feeling function, it was considered pathological. Our strong feelings were seen as a threat to the closed systems we lived in. The medical system often medicates these strong feelings. When medicated, they are numbed and disconnected from intrinsic power. This disconnects us from our real selves, the place within where our intrinsic power lies.

Since we are conditioned to disconnect from our real selves during the first half of our lives, we become frightened by our intense feelings when they surface. We begin to fear our power. When our hormones fall, our intensity rises. This is our soul's attempt to dismantle the parts that we compartmentalized in order to adapt to society's rules. In midlife, the soul asks us to deconstruct these adapted parts and reclaim those that have passion for truth and justice.

For as long as we remain disconnected from our real selves, we will be unable to transform the state of our world. We will be disconnected with our intrinsic power and feel helpless in this weakened state. We will not be able to fulfill our life's work. Women arrive at their doctor's offices hoping to find answers to explain the depth of their feelings and to learn to relate to them in new ways. They long to connect with their *real* selves that have suffered from neglect while they have been dutifully engaged in serving the needs of the world.

In a culture where fairy tales portray the sleeping princess rescued by a prince or a knight in shining armor, we are programmed to live a life of expectancy, patiently waiting for him to wake us up and rescue us from our plight. We are conditioned to feel like victims waiting to be rescued. We integrate these fairy tales into our psyches. They are really meant to help us connect with our inner parts that are symbolized by the characters portrayed. Unfortunately, our society has taught us to externalize these rather than see them as parts of ourselves. We need to internalize these characters and connect with them in order to truly feel whole. Fortunately, societal distortions break down in midlife. Reality sings a different song. Sooner or later, every woman realizes that *she* is her own "knight in shining armor." *She* is her own prince and *she* must be self-responsible for her own happiness. She needs to awaken her strong and healthy masculine energy and learn to rely on it. When the Hero and Heroine awaken inside of her, she must obey their call. Her changing hormones catalyze their awakening and she must integrate these parts into her life in order to reclaim herself and her wholeness. This requires her to live from a place of soul.

A framework that supports this journey is missing in our society and women everywhere are searching hungrily for a way to orient themselves through their midlife gateways in order to connect with what is real, true and authentic. Women are searching for ways to live from their intrinsic power. They must connect with it and empower each other to do the same. They must begin to live creatively and release their compromises that they have made from fear.

The process of empowerment

A woman's intrinsic health involves awakening to the distortions that she has been living from which abdicate her power and creativity. This awakening causes deep sorrow and disillusionment. A woman may at first feel anger and then grief. She may sometimes project this onto her partner and her family. This may startle her. She may blame her partner for her feelings of disempowerment until she realizes that *she* is responsible for reclaiming her power. She may have been conditioned to become dependent on her partner's masculine energy rather than her own. This dependency creates a movement away from her creative abilities and her intrinsic self. Her anger at the loss of connection to her real self is often projected onto her partner. She must awaken to this and use her anger creatively in order to evoke a course correction back to her true self. This course correction will awaken her inner "knight in shining armor," her masculine energy and her ability to become self-reliant and productive. This will restore her self-worth.

This is difficult, but necessary work. The more aware a woman is of losing her creative energy through anger projected on to others, the faster she will awaken her dormant and sleeping parts in her psyche. These are the parts that were dis-empowered when she lived from codependency. For as long as her worth and her value are defined by others, she will not be able to empower herself.

The unfamiliarity of feeling the connection to her real self and the familiarity of codependency in relationships create a tension inside that requires her understanding. This tension is where a woman's power gets trapped. As she begins to behave from a place that is authentic and true to herself, her new behavior gathers momentum that can redefine her from an intrinsic place. From this place, she is able to become the leader of her life and a mentor for others.

It takes great courage to connect with one's voice after having lived from the distortions of self that one is leaving behind. During midlife, many women feel deep outrage when they realize that their lives have been mostly lived in the service of others. When these others move on, women often feel lost and lose their feelings of self-worth.

Our conditioning by society disconnects us from our intrinsic power. Our feelings of resistance to perpetuating these behaviors can empower us against conforming to the "power principle." This resistance is the voice of our intrinsic power that is trying to tell us that we have compromised our truth for acceptance in society.

By the time we are in midlife, we have abdicated so much of our power to societal constructs that, like Nan, we may feel disconnected from our real selves.

Redefining intrinsic worth

In the context of performance as worth, we are not valued for who we are, but for how well we perform. This is an extrinsic measure of our worth. When we sacrifice ourselves in favor of others, we pay a price with our health. When midlife approaches, we often become ill or depressed. Our relationships may suffer until we begin to reclaim and redefine ourselves intrinsically. When we make contact with our intrinsic power, we must grieve the losses we have suffered and redefine ourselves through the language of our souls. This is a powerful and alchemical process that is often painful. It forces

186

us to create our foundations anew, based on real connections with ourselves and others.

One of the greatest lessons midlife women need to learn is how to know their limits. While caring for others at the cost of themselves, they can lose sight of their limits. Knowing their limits is difficult for women who do not have healthy boundaries. Their foundation thus far has been defined only in relationship to others. In this dynamic, women do not feel intrinsically grounded. They must begin the journey of self-discovery and reclamation, where they are able to feel what is healthy and what is not. This is a rebirth necessary for the restoration of health.

The signs of rebirth

Many of my patients become extremely anxious and depressed during their midlife transitions. This is the gateway where the language of the soul replaces the language of the world and women often feel like they are on foreign ground. The tension created between the expectations of the world and the demands of the soul provokes anxiety. A woman at this juncture needs guidance and orientation to travel from one level of identity to another. This "medial time," is the time when she has not yet embodied wholeness. First, she has much to deconstruct of her old identity that is defined by the world. This identity carries momentum and familiarity. She has to learn a new language, the language that her soul expects her to learn and understand. She has to learn how to live in the world without compromising herself. She needs to learn who she is and what makes her tick. At this juncture she may find that what is intrinsically real for her, and what she has been conditioned to believe, are different, and the chasm between them evokes anger and anxiety. This is an awakening process, one which is not marked by our culture. It is marked by her changing hormones.

Midlife women need the courage to help each other reframe this powerful time as a movement towards health. Those who have integrated their real selves into their identities must midwife those who are still in process. This is the work of the "village." We must mentor each other in order to offer orientation and direction through the treacherous terrain of this journey where our vulnerability can lead us easily back into familiar patterns of self-denial. Our new-found power may not yet have gathered momentum, and we are much like newborns in this rebirthing process. As we help each other understand the depth of our feelings and consider this process sacred, our symptoms of anxiety will be short-lived. They will be replaced with curiosity and creative fire.

The "Power Principle" in action

In the medical system, the "power principle" is prevalent in the physician-patient relationship. Physicians through their expertise, hold power over their patient's process. The patient relies on them for answers. When their feelings and stories are dismissed or medicated, they undermine themselves, and lose contact with their power. During my medical training, I often observed this in the physician-patient relationship, but I did not have a framework to understand what was happening. No matter how much I attempted to normalize it, I was unable to. As a woman who was raised in the Indian culture, I was taught that self-sacrifice was a virtue required for acceptance. As I became conditioned by this, I lost contact with my inner self. I felt intrinsic resistance to this framework, but was unable to define my resistance as a sign of health. I felt that somehow *I* was wrong for feeling it. I attempted to compensate through my performance and lost sight of my limits. This made me vulnerable to abuse by the "power principle."

Adaptation to the "power principle" was modeled for me as a noble and honorable sacrifice. The Indian culture still expects women to burn on funeral pyres in rural villages after their husbands' die, as they are considered to have no identity apart from them. The female abdicates her life and power in service of the male.

When I chose a relationship, it was through this dysfunctional framework. I found myself on familiar ground. Without a relative position, I tolerated disrespect and coped with it by working harder. I experienced deep suffering at the receiving end of the "power principle." I had no voice and no power. My self-doubt was reinforced. I found myself living in a closed system. During my recovery process, I had to reexamine all the ways that my fear had caused me to abdicate my power. I had modeled this adapted behavior to my children and was terrified they would mimic these patterns in their relationships. My awakening to this reality was painful. It was accompanied by a deep feeling of loss. I worked with this feeling until I was able to validate it. I was able to understand this loss as a result of my self-betrayal.

Through this journey, I learned how to love myself and healed my connection with my intrinsic power. I was guided by many women who had gone through similar losses before me and they midwifed my process. At first, my new-found sense of self felt vulnerable and fearful, but in time, it began to feel familiar. It defined the new me.

I realized that through this process of recovery and renewal, I had created a relative position for health for my children. They had been imprinted by my old and conditioned relationship to myself that I had replaced with a new and healthy one. This new and healthy relationship could become their secondary imprint. Because of my recovery, they could choose which one to live from. The consistency of my commitment to my real self became their comfort. They came to rely on it for strength and guidance.

Four ways in which women lose power

There are four ways in which women lose their power and lose contact with their real selves:

189

1. The wounding of instinct.

When we were young, we were told to ignore the voice of our instincts if they were in contrast to the closed system's rules. We were conditioned to obey these rules and compromised ourselves out of fear. We relied on our mentors for guidance. Many of them were also conditioned. Over time, we lost contact with our inner cues which were our feelings of resistance to what was not true for us. We lost contact with our inner wisdom, the feeling that told us that danger was near. We normalized this wounded feeling and lived from conditioned patterns even though they did not resonate with our truth.

We lost contact with our instincts. We second-guessed ourselves. For women, this pattern is epidemic. We were programmed to rely on others and to not think for ourselves. This was covertly projected onto us by the media and by society's interpretation of fairy tales. When we lost contact with our instincts, we lost contact with what was real for us. We felt unsafe. We became disempowered. We learned to give others authority over our inner wisdom and relied on their directives rather than our own. We felt powerless. We became vulnerable to abuse.

2. The wounding of feeling function.

Our feeling function is deeply wounded by society's injunctions towards it. Our strong feelings are considered pathological. In our society, passion is normalized only when it is associated with sex, but not when we feel passionately towards issues of truth and sovereignty. In this context, our passion is considered abnormal, and often necessitates medication. It causes us to feel unsafe in relationship to our strong feeling function. One of my patients described herself as having *too much* feeling. She criticized herself for this as partners in her previous relationships had left her because of this quality. They were not able to handle her passion for life and for what deeply mattered to her.

This is a serious problem in our society. A society that is afraid of deep feeling will suffer from soul loss. The feeling function is the expression of the soul, and its voice becomes louder in midlife when the soul demands to be heard through deep feelings. When we are able to have a healthy and positive relationship with our feeling function, we can become highly creative and begin to live from joy. But, without a healthy and positive framework around feelings, they become compartmentalized and we lose connection to ourselves and our souls. This results in the loss of our intrinsic power and sets us up for a negative relationship with our feeling function. We criticize ourselves when our deep feelings emerge and we apologize to others for them. This makes us vulnerable to abuse. This leaves us with feelings of emptiness and loss of meaning and an inability to experience joy. It also causes us to fear our own power.

3. The medicating of anxiety (during individuation).

Many women in midlife are in the process of individuating. They are leaving their old selves behind and birthing their new selves. These selves speak a new language—the language of feeling and meaning. Nothing less suffices. When women go through this "medial process," the separation with what is familiar and expected begins to fade and their new voice becomes louder. It keeps women up at night and speaks through their instincts and feeling function letting them know what is right and what is wrong, what is of worth and what is not. Since many women have wounded relationships with themselves, this causes them anxiety. No one has prepared them for this.

When women are medicated during this process, it threatens to interrupt their alchemical transformation. A midlife woman's anxiety is often a signal that transformation is underway and that she must direct a great amount of her energy and attention towards it. The experts she relies on may confuse the anxiety of transformation with an anxiety disorder and erroneously medicate her symptoms, interrupting her natural and powerful transformation. She must seek guidance to move through this process with the help of therapy or from those that have gone before her, and use medications during this stage with awareness and caution.

4. Relationships with each other through the "power principle" dynamic.

Many women also engage the "power principle" by trying to dominate and control others in order to feel a sense of power, control and security. This is a passive-aggressive act from their shadows which is ultimately disempowering for all. It is a covert pattern that creates distrust amongst women and deepens their wounding. Some women may mistakenly think that a way to heal their powerlessness is to take power from other women. When normalized by others, these behaviors can become regular patterns in their relationships. These patterns deepen the wounds of powerlessness in the collective feminine psyche. One of my patients awakened to this pattern in her fifties and apologized to all the women she had hurt due to it. She took responsibility for her mal-intentions towards them that arose from jealousy stemming from her lack of self-worth. In this manner, she healed her relationships with other women in addition to restoring her intrinsic power, self-respect and self-worth. In this way, she modeled her newly established integrity for others.

Anger as a sign of health

If a woman has to ask to have a need met, she is perceived as demanding, needy and dependent by others as well as herself. . . . When normal needs are denied, she begins to feel that she has no right to pursue activities that would fill her own needs and wants. Somehow she begins to expect that she has no rights at all.

~Maureen Murdock

In my own life, I learned that expressing my needs was considered selfish and unreasonable. In my former relationship, I lived in fear of having any needs at all. I felt ashamed when my needs surfaced and I tried talking myself out of them. My journals became the vehicle where I would express my confusion about having the need for love and respect and being punished for it. I was angry that I could not understand the cause for my confusion. I felt ashamed for feeling angry. This shame disconnected me from my power. I abdicated my power in order to survive.

Like Nan, I felt lost when I ended this relationship. I had difficulty making contact with my true self that was buried underneath the self that had spent half a lifetime adapting to the "power principle." I had become separated from my real self through this dynamic and was afraid to assert this self for fear that I would lose everything that I held sacred. I was convinced that my "knight in shining armor" would somehow emerge in this relationship, and I waited patiently for years. The externalized fairy tales, I believed as a child, had also directed my behavior. This "external knight," would come with a price. In my case, it was the sacrifice of my intrinsic power. I did not know any fairy tales that spoke about *my* sovereignty, or *my* will. Most of the time, I suffered in silence. I was set up for this by the "power principle." I was imprinted to believe that the virtuous path was for me to endure this treatment as a mark of a "strong woman."

My journey through midlife forced me to deconstruct this painful and disrespectful dynamic. This is not an uncommon journey for many women. The process of deconstruction and reconstruction, the death and life cycle of transformation, sometimes calls for a complete deconstruction of one's life that has been constructed around the loss of one's intrinsic power. Some women go through this process consciously while others through a crisis which leads to the dismantling of the adapted self in order for the real self to emerge. As one moves through the stages of death and life, one can feel safe again after one is able to heal the wounded instinct and re-establish boundaries that shield and protect one from harm. This shield becomes a part of one's presence and marks the initiation into mentorship.

Our life's themes

I believe our lives require us to do precise work on ourselves. We all have specific themes that unfold in our lives which we need to understand in order to live consciously. A well lived life is one lived with a consciousness of these themes, and one can seek to identify them as their life unfolds. The soul calls us to understand these themes and to live from them. The further removed we are from them, the more unfulfilled, depressed and anxious we will feel. We must awaken to the personal and transpersonal purposes of our life journeys and fulfill our sacred purpose in life. As we stay open to this framework, and look for clues and answers needed to heal our wounded parts, our real selves are more able to embody these themes more fully.

It is impossible to feel like a victim when one lives from this framework. This is one way in which our intrinsic power can be preserved. As soon as we identify with the Victim, we lose our power. Through understanding our precise purpose, we can use our biographies and our life experiences to piece together our life's themes and consciously embark on the path before us. Those who are seeking in this manner will find others who are seeking in the same manner. Their shared intentions will provide the help and support needed to stay on this path.

Imagine the field of medicine practiced with the awareness of this transformational framework. This framework is necessary in order for people to feel safe within the medical paradigm. A medical paradigm based on this framework would honor authenticity and truth and encourage patients to uncover the causes for their illnesses and despair. Through this framework, the Feminine Principle would be present in the relationships between physicians and their patients. Integrating elements of the Feminine Principle would allow physicians to support and orient their patients through their transformational journeys.

The midlife psyche

In midlife, the psyche becomes fortified to live from a level of fierceness and authenticity that surprises many women. This is a characteristic that is necessary when one is deconstructing their relationship with the "power principle." Women all over the world are going through this level of reclamation. It is a bittersweet awakening that challenges their distorted and wounded identities. They must remember that they are in the good company of others like them, and they must assert their wills in order to choose their truth. Every woman who rejects the closed system in order to create an open one by becoming real takes a step towards health and wholeness.

Archetypes in the psyche

Archetypes were defined by Carl Jung as "universal forms in the psyche that channel experiences and emotions, resulting in recognizable and typical patterns of behavior with certain probable outcomes." Archetypes can be understood through the roles they play in our lives. They exist in our psyches both in their light and shadow forms. The light form of the archetype is its representation from its higher truth. The shadow form is less connected to integrity. For example, the light form of the Magician can be expressed as a strategist in relationships for resolving conflicts or negotiating difficult interactions; the shadow form can appear as the Sorcerer that manipulates and steals power in order to dominate and control.

Other archetypes are the Hero and the Heroine, the Seductress, the Prostitute, the Victim, the Patriarch, the Matriarch, the Queen, the Warrior, and the Lover. An example of the Prostitute would be one who works in a job for financial security despite a lack of fulfillment. In this scenario, one would be engaged with the shadow archetype of the Prostitute. Working for money at the cost of fulfillment is the work of the Prostitute.

Living from shadow archetypes creates internal stress. The feeling that activates these archetypes is fear. In order to heal this, one needs to activate the Warrior in order to access a place of fearlessness and courage and find creative solutions to this dilemma. The Heroine can energize courage and integrity within the Warrior. The Warrior has the ability to inspire one to look for another job. If that isn't possible, it can access the Magician, which can transform the *experience* of the current job into one with more meaning, or it can confront the Victim that dis-empowers one into feeling powerless and help one dismantle it in order to reframe one's perspective. The Prostitute operates from fear. The Warrior, the Heroine, and the Magician operate from truth, courage and integrity.

How the victim is born within us

A common shadow archetype that is familiar to most women is the Victim. When we live from the Victim, we lose contact with our intrinsic power and feel weak and helpless. These feelings are commonly evoked by the "power principle." Over time, living from this archetype can create a pattern of behavior that disconnects us from our real selves.

The Victim renders us powerless. Due to imprinting by our fairy tales and systems, we often feel victimized due to our disconnection from our real selves. The anger resulting from this wounding has no avenue for expression. We may turn against ourselves and feel victimized by our own self-talk. Our negative self-talk shames and judges us. Many women say that they can hear their inner-critic constantly shaming them in the back of their minds. It drowns out the sound of their true voice. When they behave in accordance to the voice of the inner-critic, they unconsciously collude against themselves. Their relationships with the "power principle" often resonate with their relationship with their inner-critic. When they are dominated like this, they feel trapped. When women become aware of their inner dialogue and realize the level of shame it evokes, they can begin to observe the inner-critic through their negative self-talk and begin to dismantle it. This journey is the beginning of their recovery and once they begin to heal, they are unable to tolerate abuse from the "power principle." They begin to identify more with the Warrior who can align them with the Queen and connect them with their intrinsic power.

The power of a healthy community

It is important for us to empower each other and to mirror back the power we see in each other. When we lose contact with our intrinsic power, it can help to have it reflected back to us by another. The symbol for the female is Venus' mirror (♀). It is the mirror we hold up to the other to reflect back to them their own strength. We owe it to each other to mirror back who we know is buried beneath the Victim. The Queen resides there in her power, and she often needs to be evoked and activated. Once we can access her, we can help others do the same.

The danger of a disempowered woman

Women also compete with each other for power. Such women are not connected with their intrinsic power. They may covertly sabotage the efforts of other women, while presenting the *illusion* of support. They may also avoid being in relationships with empowered women. When one is in the presence of such women, one feels unsafe. This feeling warns one of danger as one is in the presence of the "power principle" in action. Since their conscious and unconscious intentions are not in the other's best interest, they cannot be trusted. The feeling function will resist them. It must be trusted.

This shadow relationship between women is called "the dark sisterhood" pattern. It is a relationship dynamic marked by behaviors that operate from jealousy, competition and domination. Unfortunately for women, this is all too common in our society. Since many women feel disempowered, they operate from the dark sisterhood pattern in attempts to take power from other women who they feel may pose a threat. Empowered women's connection with their intrinsic power poses a threat to the self-worth of dark sisters. Dark sisters compete with healthy, empowered women in attempts to take their power in order to compensate for their own lack of self-worth. These patterns damage their relationships with other women and may also cause shame and regret within "dark sisters" because they lack integrity. What they need to understand is that relationships with empowered women can help them heal their wounded self-worth. When an empowered woman has the courage to confront a dark sister, it can help the dark sister heal the wounded relationship with herself and restore her integrity by bringing her awareness to these shadow patterns.

Many women going through midlife transformation find that the women that they thought were their friends leave their lives when they connect to their intrinsic power. These friends will not resonate with the woman who is transforming into her real self unless they have transformed themselves. It is imperative to be able to identify and name this unhealthy behavior, and to dismantle unhealthy relationships that are disempowering. The danger of staying in relationships that operate from this dynamic is that they can hold us back in our process and sabotage our ability to activate the Queen. Many women who are recalibrating their lives feel loyalty to the friends they are leaving behind. They struggle with the loss of these friendships when they lose resonance with them during transformation. They need to trust that relationships that are healthy and committed to growth will remain, but the unhealthy ones need to fall away. They must grieve these losses and continue on the path towards becoming real.

The danger of self-doubt

Self-doubt is a hook that causes us to identify with the Victim archetype. As victims, we are not connected to our power, but feel a sense of power through blaming others for our plights. The Victim weakens our Energy body. It causes loss of vitality and creativity. Sometimes it can sabotage our access to the Heroine and the Warrior which are archetypes needed for us to awaken the Magician and the Queen. We must engage our strength and not allow our grief from loss of relationships to activate our self-doubt. This can sabotage our forward movement that is necessary for our *true* healing.

As our current paradigm shifts from competition to collaboration, we must identify the core values within the open system that it can become. We must include ways of supporting one another authentically with elements of the Feminine Principle.

Nan revisited

Nan was fully engaged with her Victim archetype. She wanted someone to do something *for* her, so she could live out the life familiar to her. She was looking for hormone replacement therapy or a hysterectomy to free her from her plight. I could have easily taken the bait and capitulated as her rescuer. I had the training to fix her symptoms, but if I did that without engaging her process, she would not be able to connect with her intrinsic power.

In her current state, she felt like a victim of her changing body.

She lost contact with her inner limits of satiety and avoided her reflection in the mirror. If she had seen herself grow obese, she could have awakened self-responsibility and confronted the Victim with the Warrior or the Heroine. She had been conditioned to rely on the expectations of others around her. At this point, she perceived me as her "knight in shining armor." If I had capitulated to her pleas, I could have operated as the knight on her behalf. This would have held her hostage in her Victim and she would have missed the opportunity to catalyze her process of contacting her soul, where her feminine power resided. Her power would have remained buried underneath the layers of adaptation and conditioning where it would have built pressure in her Energy and Emotional bodies, waiting for a crisis to release it.

Midlife as a transformative individuation process

Joseph Campbell states in his book, *The Hero with a Thousand Faces*, that if the opportunity to use the catalytic energy of transformation is missed, life loses its sense of meaning and one lives out of the "wasteland" as a victim.

Many people in our society have missed the opportunity to unfold an authentic life because of the lack of framework in our health care system available for guidance during this powerful and transformational time. In order for us to truly heal, we must reframe how we define health to restore our connection with the parts essential for activating our true selves. A prescription drug cannot accomplish this. Only a framework that empowers us to explore our life themes and to live from them during the second half of our lives can help us with this sacred task.

In the middle of our lives, we have all reached the half-way point. This is often marked by a woman's physiological changes and by her feelings of anger, resistance, depression and anxiety. Her hot flashes and night sweats—although symptoms of hormonal change—are also indicators of a time in her life when the call from her soul is the loudest. It asks her to evaluate if she is living from her intrinsic power and if she is being true to herself. If she is not, she must seek out and journey to understand herself and resist the temptation for becoming a victim. She must find her voice, her truth and her power, and she must gather her courage to stand at this gateway and allow herself to reconstruct her life from a place of inner truth. Her menopausal symptoms may mark the threshold where her psyche begins to speak the loudest and her feeling function is recovering its voice. If she fails to consider this as a transformational time and feels victimized by it, then she will subject herself to great peril. The wasteland will await her meaningless existence where she will continue to play out her roles to please the world. Her soul will inevitably speak through the presentation of her fate in its ever loving faithfulness to offer her the opportunity to transform. This will be her "midlife crisis." She will be called here to arise out of the Victim by evoking the Heroine and the Warrior in order to activate the Magician and connect with the Queen. This initiation will be needed for her to reclaim her power and mentor others.

If our society embodied this framework, it could transform into one that valued the midlife journey. In a society like this, we could live the second half of our lives fulfilled and satisfied as a result of our well-lived lives, and we could die fearless deaths. Our lives could be a testament to the mythic process that regarded initiation and individuation as sacred passages. Many cultures consider the start and cessation of menses as initiations into different phases of women's lives. These are deeply sacred rites of passages. They must be marked and honored as opportunities for deeper awakening and empowerment, not as the "curses" they are currently considered.

Because my wake-up call came as a deep betrayal of all that I held sacred, this held the precise "medicine" for my reclamation. To the degree that I had given over my power to the other, I had the opportunity to reclaim it and to reconnect to my authentic self. I utilized a multitude of healers whom I relied on to reflect my true self back to me. Their facilitation offered me a safe space for my Four Bodies to align with my real self. This process was deeply terrifying but also deeply powerful. As I began to hear my own voice underneath the injunctions of my conditioning, I began to feel alive and learned to feel comfortable with my intrinsic power. I channeled my energy into reconstructing my life from a place that was real and free from fear. I learned how to hold sacred space for my patients who were transforming like I was. I felt a responsibility to pay this gift forward to others. Those of us who survive the midlife gateway and reconstruct our lives anew have a responsibility to be present for others in the same way our mentors have been for us.

As far as Nan, she learned how to feel safe in her process by understanding the terrain of transformation. She slowly began to uncover the voice of her inner critic who was victimizing her. She began to make better food choices, take walks, journal, attend art classes, record her dreams and work with me to balance her hormones. Over a three month period, she began to grieve the loss of herself and recognized her conditioned patterns as compromises of her truth. She learned to understand and connect with her feeling function in therapy. She used acupuncture to regain her vitality, and body work to release the stress in her muscles, and she began to reorient and reframe her relationship to herself. She became aware of how her body felt. She began to feel sensations in her body again, the sensation of her breath when she exercised, and how food tasted in her mouth. She also began to notice when she felt full. She stopped drinking to relax. She found it numbed her senses and as a result, her hot flashes improved. She began to look at herself in the mirror. Within a year, she had lost 65 pounds and was well on her way to a vital and more meaningful life that resonated with her soul. She worked with a psychotherapist, and through much reflection decided to become a massage therapist. It was her way of "paying forward" the wisdom and insight she received during her transformational process. Her libido recovered and her bleeding was no longer heavy. She had a new lease on life, a new understanding of herself and a new connection to her intrinsic power. She formed a new dialogue with herself that reminded her to stay connected with her truth. She dismantled the inner critic who had dominated her life. She encountered her Warrior and Heroine who awakened her Magician. The weepy, victimized woman I met a year ago morphed into a powerful and beautiful midlife woman who now understands the precision of life and trusts in the process of transformation. She is well on her way to awakening the Queen and becoming a mentor for others.

8

Reclaiming the Feminine

Flight

As I break open,
I uncover forbidden secrets,
They fly out from dark places fluttering
like butterflies in the sun.
My soul heaves an exhale,
lightened from releasing
the oppressive weight of misogyny.
With this lightened,
I transform;
and like bud to blossom,
turn my face to the Sun.
I can now flap my wings
and take flight.

The most powerful word spoken by a woman is "NO."

~Rose Kumar, M.D.

What is the feminine? The answer to this question needs purification and clarity. She has been defined by our systems, our fairy tales and advertisements. We have attempted to embody her definition in the ways that we look and behave. She is imprinted in our psyches with a physical appearance that is unattainable for most. We neglect to value her intrinsic power and strength. Instead, we glorify her appearance and distort who she really is. Through society's lens she is portrayed as large breasted with full lips and a boundless sex drive. She doesn't speak, and when she does, she says what is expected in order to keep the peace. She follows the system's rules with her silence. These rules define the conduct she must follow to earn the label of a "good girl." She normalizes what is unhealthy in order to feel "loved." She keeps her truth hidden in her throat and her heart, afraid of being punished for speaking it.

We all participate in defining the feminine through what we buy, what we watch and what we enable. We mentor this feminine image to our children and imprint them with our embodiment of her. We have stereotyped her into an unattainable figure that never ages. She only feels what society tells her to feel. She doesn't emote and she doesn't rock the boat. She is the primadonna who adapts and yields.

One of my midlife patients described her mother as a "saint." Her father was an abusive and dominating alcoholic and her mother kept her mouth shut. She bore his abuse saying nothing. She thought that her mother's strength was a noble feat deserving of sainthood. She had a difficult life after she left home and struggled with her inner demons. I asked her to consider what it would have been like if her mother had spoken up against the abuse to protect herself and her children with sovereignty, and *not* normalized her father's behavior. Maybe she wouldn't have spent so much of her life recreating what felt familiar. In speaking up, her mother could have modeled a relative position for health that would have given her children the opportunity to make healthier choices in their lives. She realized that her definition of sainthood was influenced by how society viewed women who tolerated abuse. Through a healthier lens, she had a different definition of strength and was able to redefine sainthood.

Cathy

Cathy is a 49-year-old woman who came to see me with complaints of irritable bowel syndrome (IBS). She had frequent abdominal cramps, was unable to have normal bowels movements, and knew where a bathroom was in every store. In addition to IBS, she felt hot and cold throughout the day. She believed she emotionally overreacted in relationships so she isolated herself from others to save *them* from her agitation. She suffered from chronic fatigue and became progressively home bound. She ate to comfort herself and, gradually, her life lost its meaning. Her menstrual cycles were irregular and she was unable to sleep through the night. Every day she felt like her life was wasting away. She was a homemaker and had two teenage children. Her husband, Bill, was an executive. Economic pressures burdened him with stress and long hours at work. He was hypertensive, had elevated cholesterol and was moderately obese.

After work, Bill would want to rest in order to release stress from the day. Cathy was not able to keep a clean house due to her symptoms, and looked forward to his arrival which abated her isolation and loneliness. Bill would drink a few martinis to "relax" and then he would let his emotions loose. Cathy's evenings were ultimately spent in "survival mode." She felt ashamed for not being able to keep a clean house. Her teenage children offered no help. She felt alone and isolated. She felt like she was drowning from the expectations put upon her in addition to her physical symptoms.

Cathy and Bill had been married for seventeen years. They decided to achieve the "American dream." This was their goal since their twenties. They were willing to make the needed sacrifices for it. Now in their forties, they had a big house, a fancy car, an executive job, social status and most of the material possessions that defined their dream. They had sacrificed the time needed to cultivate their relationships with each other and their family. They were preoccupied with achieving the social definition of success. Neither Cathy nor Bill really knew their children. They were busy achieving their goals at the cost of their relationships.

At 47, Cathy felt that her life was passing her by. She had gained 50 pounds, and did not feel well. When she came to see me, she was on five medications: two for depression, one for abdominal pain, one for insomnia and one for anxiety. None were working. Her physician dismissed her, as he was unable to fix her symptoms. He had tripled her dose of antidepressants in the past six months because they were ineffective. Since then, she told me she could not feel empathy. She said she felt flat and numb.

Cathy was also caught in a pattern of fight-or-flight. In her forties, she became more sensitive to her husband's behavior. She grew agitated an hour before he got home, anticipating his drinking and abuse pattern that demeaned and shamed her. She would tremble before his arrival. She remembered the times when they were first married. They enjoyed two years of bliss, and then he was gone, spending long hours at work. She was pregnant and decided to stay home to raise children and play the role of the executive's wife.

Our culture associates success with high performance and financial status. This is defined by how much money we make and what that money can buy. Our big homes become symbols of our success and our expensive cars mark our position in society. We become consumers. We shop, we drink, and we eat rich foods. We normalize these behaviors and associate them with success. The cultural motto we serve is—the bigger the better, the more the better, the faster the better, the richer the better.

We lose our sight of the fact that life is a journey, a process. We miss the meaning in our lives and feel emptiness, but continue our patterns without attending to our feelings. When we arrive in midlife feeling this way, our emptiness cannot be healed with medications. It is a symptom of the life that we have missed. It may manifest as anxiety or depression, IBS or hypertension; it may manifest as an addiction or a heart attack. We have sacrificed *process* for *product*. It is time for us move inward and redefine ourselves.

The Masculine and Feminine Principles

The East offers a perspective that sees wholeness as a complete circle. This circle consists of two halves, Yin and Yang. The energies of both are intrinsic to life and health. When they are imbalanced, we become sick. When they are balanced, we feel whole. Neither is associated with gender and men and women have energies of both within them. These energies are also present in nature and food and as characteristics in our behaviors. The concept of "process versus product" can be applied to an even larger perspective of wholeness. This perspective considers that our behaviors contain elements of both Feminine and Masculine Principles as well as elements of Yin and Yang energies. Emphasizing elements of one over the other can lead to imbalance. Being aware of this larger perspective of wholeness and the energies that are contained within it, can make us conscious of how we live and relate to one another.

The Masculine Principle is defined by characteristics such as linear and rational thinking, analytical thinking, doing, light, product or outcome focus, action oriented, external or outward focus, fast and quick, ego, mental focus, competitive and "either or" oriented. It contains the qualities of heat. It contains the Yang energy.

The Feminine Principle includes characteristics such as cyclical, non-rational, strategic thinking, dark, process orientated, inward or internal focus, being, intuitive, creative, receptive, feeling, patient, heart and soul identified, collaborative and 'both and' oriented. It contains the qualities of coolness. It contains the Yin energy.

Society glorifies only elements of the Masculine Principle. We

THE MASCULINE PRINCIPLE	THE FEMININE PRINCIPLE
linear	cyclical
analytical	strategic
mental	feeling
fast/quick	slow
light	dark
active	receptive
either/or	both/and
doing	being
product/outcome oriented	process oriented
external focus	internal focus
competitive	collaborative
rational	non-rational/intuitive
hot	cool
Yang	Yin
fixing	healing
manifesting	incubating

Figure 7: Elements of the Masculine and Feminine Principles

are valued and rewarded more when we live from these elements rather than those of the Feminine Principle. When we are product oriented, rational and analytical in our thinking, we are considered "team players" and assets to our jobs. Our society does not value creativity, an element of the Feminine Principle, to the same degree. It has been dismantled from our education and health care systems. We are expected to think "inside the box." Anything outside of it is discarded. The Masculine Principle, at the cost of the Feminine, leaves us unbalanced and unhealthy.

Both men and women have associated success and worth with the elements of the Masculine Principle. Cathy and Bill were so

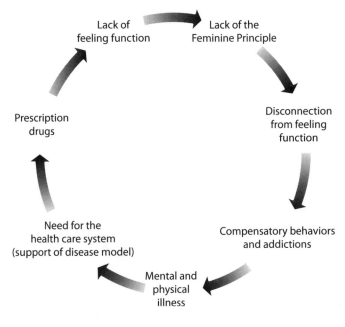

Figure 8: Lack of the Feminine Principle

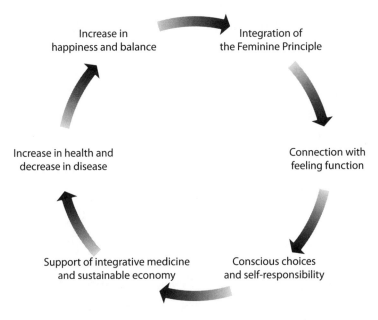

Figure 9: Integration of the Feminine Principle

busy achieving (doing) the material dream (product) that they failed to spend time with their family (being). The *process* of life had less importance to them than the *product* of life. It led to ill-health and lack of fulfillment. They arrived in their forties symptomatic and without real meaning.

If we look at what our society values, we can see that it is largely the Masculine Principle. Our bonuses and worth are based on productivity. We strive to make money at any cost. This is glorified in our movies and television shows. We devalue process and value product. Analytical, not creative, thinking is rewarded. If we are creative, kinesthetic, artistic or sensitive then we do not fit in. Our society undervalues these gifts. We are expected to suppress them. We compromise who we really are and bury our feminine qualities in favor of those identified with the Masculine Principle.

Our culture has become so obsessed with this external definition of worth that people go into credit card debt in order to project the illusion of success. This is not sustainable. It is not even honest. Eventually, we have to confront ourselves in order to live from a place that is real and not illusory. The real place within, is one that always moves towards wholeness. The Masculine and Feminine Principles are balanced here.

Our medical culture is no different in its emphasis of the Masculine Principle. It glorifies its elements. Fixing, focus on outcomes and analytical thinking are valued over the feminine elements of listening, creative problem solving, intuiting, collaborating and process. We use terms like "war on cancer," "attack on heart disease" and "survival" rather than seeking and healing. In relationship to the medical system, patients feel like victims who can be rescued by the experts. Instincts and intuitions currently have no place and are ignored by both patients and physicians. If the experts cannot fix them, patients give up on themselves and sometimes on life itself. They are unable to access wholeness. They live out the prognoses predicted for them. Illness is not considered a journey or a process by our medical system. Patients are not supported in their exploration of answers. They are left to do this alone with their looming doubts and fears, believing their personal process does not hold credibility; rather credibility lies in the hands of the experts.

The price of the "quick fix"

In the sixties when medicine became quick-fix oriented, it deeply influenced our culture. It enabled complacency and cultivated a cultural mindset that sought quick-fixes only to remedy symptoms. This became the mindset that we applied to many areas of life. Our emphasis is still on quick-fixes, not on self-responsibility for well-*being*. This has cost us greatly and has enabled the escalation of industries that profit from the production of (synthetic) medications. Most of these numb our feeling function. Other cultures are not as imbalanced as we are. They value elements of the Feminine Principle. They value feelings. This is reflected in their state of health which is far better than ours.

Inner work requires labor. Labor is time and effort intensive. It does not rely on quick-fixes. It requires strategy and insight and examines causes carefully. It does not shirk from hardship. It endures and has tenacity. It is resilient and patient. It is transforming, transmuting and regenerative. This feels counterintuitive to our quick-fix mentality as this works against the momentum of our normalized cultural construct. It takes added effort on our parts to cultivate well-being. If we are not aware, there is danger that we will join the path of least resistance and settle for quick-fixes.

The quick-fix mentality has had a significant impact on our personal health, as well as, on the cost of health care in this country. People in the U.S. are realizing that traditional medicine operates from only half of the circle of wholeness. Without elements of the Feminine Principle, it is unable to provide *true* healing. The linear focus of the Masculine Principle needs the intuitive focus of the

Feminine Principle for wholeness. The imbalance in our system manifests in patient disillusionment and is also reflected in the rising costs of malpractice insurance. Most cases of malpractice are a result of the neglected Feminine Principle in the physician-patient encounter. Listening is crucial to formulating a correct diagnosis. In a patient visit that is valued for its speed by corporate health care, physicians are unable to devote the time needed for listening to patient histories with their full attention. When they miss crucial clues needed to diagnose and treat, they often make mistakes in medical judgment. Both patients and physicians suffer needless wounding in this way. The absence of the Feminine Principle in health care leads to stress and burnout amongst physicians. We all pay a price for this. Our medical system needs to function from both the Feminine and Masculine Principles in order to be healthy and whole and to effectively serve all of its participants including its physicians and patients.

Like Cathy, many women become disconnected from the Feminine Principle in both their inner and outer worlds. When we were children, we lived almost exclusively from the Feminine Principle. We lived in a world of imagination, beauty and creativity. As we aged and became socialized and conditioned, our worth became identified with more elements of the Masculine Principle. We learned to override our feeling function and instincts in favor of thinking. We separated from our authentic selves without realizing it.

Women have an active Emotional body and strong feeling function. Our feeling function is one of our greatest gifts. It is always trying to bring us into a state of wholeness by activating the Emotional body. When we begin to connect with our feeling function, we begin to heal. Women who heal in midlife have reintegrated elements of the Feminine Principle into their lives. They find value in self-care. For many, their journeys involve a deep exploration of their Four Body System and through this, a reconnection with their real selves. They are able to uncover areas of imbalance caused by self-neglect that call for healing and transformation. Without these efforts, they can never live from wholeness.

Patty

Patty is a 43-year-old woman who had a long journey with infertility. Between the ages of 34 and 36, she had gone through four cycles of in vitro fertilization without success. During this time, she felt stress and shame for not being able to conceive and felt inadequate as a woman.

Six months after she stopped treatments, she became pregnant. After her baby was born, she began to experience chronic anxiety triggered by financial stress. She began to have a recurring dream about suffocating. In the dream she was surrounded by smoke and had trouble breathing. She felt that she was unable to see through the smoke into her future, and she would frequently wake up in a state of panic. She was living from the fight-or-flight response every day and had no control over it. Over the past few years, she felt more agitated and overwhelmed even when under mild amounts of stress. The feelings of inadequacy she experienced during the infertility treatments returned. She began to feel shame and anger towards herself and she felt like she was reliving that stressful time. She was desperate for healing.

As we worked together, she began to address the constitutional imbalances in her Energy body that resulted from performance anxiety that were returning for release. She worked with a classical homeopath to balance her constitution. Her feelings of shame needed to heal and she needed a framework in order to be able to relate to them. She was frightened about what her future held and she couldn't see herself in it, hence the smoke in her dream. Her future felt unpredictable. This was triggered by the financial stress she was under. During several Reiki sessions, she sobbed deeply and released the internal pressure from her unprocessed shame activated by the infertility treatments. This had created an imbalance in her Energy body. She brought this to consciousness in the safe space held by her therapist, and she was finally able to understand and release it. She began to learn a new language of compassion towards herself. It was the language of self-love and forgiveness.

She started to feel comfortable in her own skin. It was no longer the unsafe place of blame and shame. She felt she was learning about the parts of her that frequently felt abused by her critical self-talk and she needed to release the sorrow that this had caused within her. She was relieved to know this was a stage in her process towards wholeness. Within a month, her anxiety had healed and she felt more grounded. Her recurrent dream did not return. She slept more soundly. She felt a lightness of being and was no longer in fight-or-flight. She moved inward and worked through her transformation with guidance from her practitioners. This took a great level of courage.

Patty felt more confidence as she connected with her intrinsic power. She realized how she had devalued herself as a woman due to her social programming which surfaced during the infertility treat-ments. Although she became pregnant on her own, she was not able to acknowledge this as a sign of fertility. Her inner-critic dismissed her natural pregnancy and attributed it to chance and luck, not to her intrinsic ability to conceive. She worked hard to replace her old critical self-talk with self-acknowledgement. Patty was able to redefine herself and her worth from an intrinsic place. She experienced the power of her feeling function and its ability to connect her to increased feelings of self-worth. Through this process, her anxiety healed.

For Cathy, the process was more complex. She needed to evaluate the neglected elements of the Feminine Principle in her relation-ship to herself, as well as towards her family system. This process took over a year with her husband's participation. Through therapy, Cathy and Bill were able to identify the areas in their marriage that they sacrificed in favor of financial success. They healed their fear of financial loss by working through their issues of scarcity. Cathy began to see how her fight-or-flight response resulted from her negative self-talk that supported Bill's criticism. She realized that if she did not agree with him, she could express her feelings to him. In the past, his critic and her shame colluded with one another, causing her to spiral into low self-worth, creating stress that further imbalanced her hormones and aggravated her symptoms of IBS.

When the possibility of a healthier future became evident, she was able to choose differently from a place of self-validation and empowerment and she and Bill worked hard to change their dynamics. I helped bring balance to her hormones and showed her how to make lifestyle choices to restore her physical health. She was able to slowly wean off her medications. In seven months, she was medication free and twenty pounds lighter. Her IBS had healed and she decided to volunteer at a local nursing home by reading to the elderly. She felt that she was making a more meaningful contribution in her life. She and Bill began spending more time together. Their family took their first vacation in five years. It was the best time that they had ever had together. She had connected to her real self and could now access joy in her relationships. She learned how to fill herself up first and then overflow onto others. In addition, she implemented her lifestyle changes in her family. As a result, Bill lost forty pounds and no longer needed medications. Cathy's will to heal herself also healed her family. This is an example of the power that the Feminine Principle can have on one's health and well-being.

The body's attempt to restore balance

The Feminine Principle is as necessary for us to identify with for *process,* as the Maslive a life that is balanced with elements from *both* principles. Taking time for *being* is as important as taking time for *doing.* It is regenerative to our bodies, our minds and spirits. Research in psychoneuroimmunology has shown that living from both principles supports our immune systems.

Both Patty and Cathy needed to balance their Energy and Emotional bodies. Their Physical bodies catalyzed their process of awakening. Their Physical and Mental bodies were symptomatic. This is common in midlife. The perimenopausal and menopausal process will always bring our attention to the neglected elements of the Feminine Principle in our lives. Our bodies will call us within through symptoms and sickness in order for us to heal the areas of neglect and recalibrate ourselves with a new language of self-care and self-respect. When we do this courageous work, we can heal; when we don't, our unhealed lives express themselves through "disease." Hidden in every disease is the opportunity for us to understand the energetic imbalances that caused it.

The wounded masculine

Just as we are collectively living from the wounded feminine, we are also living from the wounded masculine. The wounded masculine identifies with the "power principle" and attempts to dominate others in order to compensate for its lack of power. This energy does not contain intrinsic power or balance. This energy is identified with domination and values competition in favor of collaboration. In our culture, the wounded masculine is normalized and glorified. Our drive for material success at the cost of process and for fixing at the cost of healing causes us grave suffering. In order for us to be whole, we all need to heal both the wounded masculine and feminine within. This is urgent and imperative in order for us to connect with our real selves.

Just as women need to live from their sovereignty independent of men, men need to live from their sovereignty independent of women. Healthy relationships are independent, yet collaborative. We need to redefine our selfhood through the Feminine and Masculine Principles and reintegrate them into our behaved lives in order to be authentic and not compensated.

Feeling function

Our feeling function is the part closest to our souls. Deep feelings threaten our sentimental society that becomes bewildered and uncomfortable around their expression. When their hormones change and the Energy and Emotional bodies release their pressure, women can become overwhelmed, and not understand the intensity of their feelings. This frightens many women. If their feelings are validated and considered normal, women are able to release and free their repressed energy. Many do this through art. Others do this through music or dance. Some do it through exercise, and some cry for months. Whatever way a woman chooses to release is the correct way. She must cleanse her system in order to regain balance. Through this process, she can make contact with her soul and her strength and learn about her Emotional body, sometimes, for the first time in her life. "Good girls don't cry" is not a healthy injunction. Good girls express their feelings. These girls are healthy.

Our feelings are never wrong. They always have a good reason for being, and understanding this allows a woman to come into a relationship with herself through self-love. It is here that she can acknowledge her soulfulness when she feels deeply and intensely. We need more of this in our culture. Trusting in our feeling function is the only way we can repair and reweave our wounded instincts and intuitions. These are the parts of us that keep us safe and sovereign. Without their protection, we remain vulnerable. When we are guided by them, we stay on course in our lives.

Midlife often awakens us and evokes our journeys back to ourselves. Many women have expressed their anguish over the discovery that they have surrounded themselves with superficial relationships which are deeply unfulfilling. Women begin to feel a lack of resonance with the people in their lives to whom they can no longer relate. Dismantling these relationships is painful, but they must reevaluate their values and dismantle everything that feels inauthentic. From this place, they can begin to trust what is real and find their voices. This deep transformation is purifying.

Many women reach this gateway in midlife and choose to not walk through it. Familiarity holds too much momentum, and they are not able or willing to engage their Warrior to purify their lives. They may slip back into what is familiar and superficial. They risk feeling like victims and look to others in order to rescue them. These women are disconnected with the truth of their real selves. They are deeply wounded. They are difficult to be in relationships with because they look to others to compensate for their lack of intrinsic power. They substitute sentimentality for love. Sentimentality masquerades as true feeling, but it isn't. The real self cannot be fooled. It will eventually call us from within. We must heed its call.

Discerning the difference between reality and illusion can be difficult if one lives a compensated life. Compensations become the familiar pattern of living, and truth feels unfamiliar. It is important for us to open our inner-eyes through our feeling function to be able to integrate the truth of who we are into our behaviors, and not settle for what may feel familiar. The longer we are able to do this, the more momentum it will carry. This pattern can soon become the new, familiar and normal one.

How to relate to one's inner critic

When we begin to transition through menopause and transform our relationships into more authentic ones, the inner-critic's voice can become very loud. Many times it will manifest through our feelings. If we feel shame or guilt during this process, we must stay aware that the inner-critic may be dialoguing with us through its familiar language. It often activates our feelings in painful ways. If we heed its directive, it can make us depressed. We are also more likely to sabotage our healing process. Some women agonize over how to stop the inner-critic's chatter. They have difficulty thinking from a place of truth as the inner-critic's voice overshadows any efforts that they may engage in order to quiet it. They may medicate themselves in various ways attempting to find inner peace, but to no avail.

A strategy that is often effective here is the practice of Mindfulness. Becoming mindful of the inner-critic's method of dialoguing can remove us from identifying with it. When we *observe* the chatter in our minds, the inner-critic cannot engage us to the degree that identifying with it can. Becoming an observer creates a separation between women and their critical self-talk. As small as this separation may initially be, it is the entry point for identifying with the *observer* of the inner-critic rather than with the inner-critic itself. In time, this separation between self and inner-critic becomes wider. This protects us from engaging the Victim and preserves our relationship with our real selves. In this way, the inner-critic's directive can become less connected to our feeling function. It may continue to try to shame a woman, but its language does not land as easily or deeply within her Emotional body. Women begin to feel a sense of freedom and regain their vitality. They no longer need to self-medicate. They feel more empowered and can create a new language for their inner dialogue. They begin to feel self-compassion and treat themselves with more respect. This brings them peace. When Mindfulness is integrated as a strategic tool in midlife, it can settle the mind and support the individuation process.

A direct dialogue with the inner-critic is usually futile. Its script is imprinted and has momentum from our life history that has been reinforced by society. When we allow the critic to victimize us, we lose our power.

Over time, as a woman engages with her real self, she begins to resonate more with her truth than with her compensated self and begins to form a new identity that is resonant with what is real for her. She develops the ability to speak her truth and is not as

221

concerned about how others view her. She becomes less adapted and more authentic. This becomes her new normal and sets her life on a course correction. This is a deeper level of her individuation.

Liz

Liz is a 42-year-old woman with three children below the ages of twelve. She has been married for thirteen years. She tolerated emotional abuse in her marriage for years. Her history revealed abuse from her mother when she was a child, where she was unable to speak her truth and was expected to stay silent in order to "keep the peace." She felt the familiarity of her family of origin when she met her husband and thought that her love could change his behavior. It didn't. When she turned forty, something inside Liz grew restless. In her deepest self, she felt a lack of resonance with her husband. When she came to see me, she suffered from insomnia and depression. She also had symptoms of acid reflux and frequently got sick when her children were. She was impatient and irritable with them. She did not know how to change this dynamic.

She had adrenal burnout and was chronically fatigued from the dynamics in her home. Her immune system was weak and vulnerable. I helped guide her with dietary changes to revive her vitality. She began receiving acupuncture treatments to restore her energy and treat her reflux. A month later, her symptoms began to improve.

She was referred to a psychotherapist and learned that she had been adapting to emotional abuse through learned helplessness. Since being shamed was a familiar pattern since childhood, she accommodated her husband's treatment without question. She had "learned" to feel helpless as a child and was unable to advocate for herself in her marital relationship as an adult.

It was only when her hormones began to change that she was unable to tolerate her husband's abuse. She felt the tension between her familiar adaptations and her new intolerance to his behavior.

This caused her considerable stress. She started to feel anger which she would then project onto her children. When she understood her patterns, she began to work to reconfigure them from a different level of self-worth. She learned how she *deserved* to be treated and began to advocate for herself to her husband.

Six months after she came to see me, she had a healthier relationship with herself. She was able to discern the dialogue of her inner-critic from the one communicated through abuse from her husband. She decided that if her husband continued to treat her with disrespect and dishonor, she would file for divorce. She knew she had the ability to do this. She began to sleep more soundly and her reflux and depression healed. She had reclaimed herself from her familiar script and connected to her intrinsic power. She no longer felt helpless. Liz discovered how learned helplessness had disconnected her from her intrinsic power and this disconnection manifested in her symptoms. She had needed to uncover her childhood patterns that had imprinted her in order to dismantle them. This changed her relationship to herself and with what she was willing to tolerate. She emerged, more empowered, through her midlife gateway.

The alchemical process of midlife

This is an ongoing journey that we all must take, one that propels us from the Victim into a self-responsible adult. The tension between the old script and our new behavior that is based in self-respect is necessary and lifesaving. Our patterns can transform only through a change in our behaviors. This has the power to undo the damage from our mental constructs as we leave our identifications with them, straddling the unknown between the self-critic and self-love. This is the powerful medial place that contains the tension of opposites. In this tension lies the catalyst we can use to make the alchemical shifts needed to become our true and real selves.

The power of "No"

It is worth repeating that the most powerful word a woman can say is, "no." When spoken with conviction and sovereignty, it has the ability to change our world as we know it. It takes great courage to say "no." We risk being rejected and abandoned. We need to remind ourselves that even when we stand alone, we are not really alone. We are in the company of our souls, our integrity and our truth. "No" activates the powerful repair work of reclamation. As we say "no" to others and behave in accordance with our instincts, we often find ourselves re-empowered and aligned with our truth. Saying "no" also activates the Hero and the Warrior who help us reconfigure our lives.

We must value "no" as a sacred word, and learn to say it when directed by our feeling function. It is a word that can initiate us into connecting with our souls. It draws the line that becomes our boundary that protects us and keeps us safe. This connects us with the Queen. In time, the Queen becomes integrated into our presence. Our sovereign presence embodies our integrity. When we say "no," we can restore our will and our worth. We are then able to assert our will in our relationship to the inner-critic and find the ability to stand strong in the tension between familiarity and freedom in our transformational process.

We must begin our awakening to what is real. "No" is a good place to start. We need to remember we always have a choice. We can choose to adapt to the societal norms of the wounded masculine and feminine, or we can choose healthy versions of these. Saying no to distortions is a choice, but this choice requires consciousness. Unless we can understand the patterns that lead to illness and lack of meaning, it is difficult for us to dismantle them. Any movement away from the norm creates tension in our system. We need the courage and endurance to maintain our position of health.

A Woman of Wisdom and a Man with Heart

The power of choice is illustrated in this powerful story of Gawain and Lady Ragnell. This is an English tale that portrays the healing of both the wounded masculine and feminine. This story takes place in fourteenth century England. I first came across it in the landmark book by Maureen Murdock called *The Heroine's Journey*.

One day in late summer, Gawain, the nephew of King Arthur was with his uncle and his knights. One day, the king returned from a day of hunting and looked visibly shaken. Gawain followed him into his chambers to ask him what had happened.

While he was out hunting, Arthur had been accosted by a fearsome knight, named Sir Gromer, who sought revenge for the loss of his lands. He spared Arthur by giving him a chance to save his life by meeting him in a year at the same spot unarmed with the correct answer to the question, "What is it that women most desire above all else?" If he found the correct answer to this question, his life would be spared.

Gawain assured Arthur that together they would be able to find the correct answer to the question and during the next year, they collected answers from near and far. As the day drew near, Arthur was worried that none of the answers held the truth.

A few days before he was to meet Gromer, Arthur journeyed out to a grove of great oaks. There before him was a large grotesque woman. She was large in length and breadth and her head was mottled green and her hair was spiked with weed like protuberances and she appeared monstrous. Her name was Lady Ragnell.

Lady Ragnell told Arthur that she was on her way to meet her stepbrother, Sir Gromer, and he did not have the right answer to the question. She told him that she knew the correct answer and that she would tell it to him if Sir Gawain would agree to marry her. Arthur cried out that he couldn't do that to Gawain.

She said that she did not ask Arthur for his agreement. She wanted to see if Gawain would himself choose to marry her. "These are my terms." She told him that she would meet him at the same spot the next day, and she disappeared into the oak grove.

Arthur was disheartened because he could not imagine his nephew marrying this hideous creature in order to save Arthur's life. Gawain saw the pale and strained look on Arthur's face and he asked him what had happened. When he told Gawain about Lady Ragnell's proposal, Gawain was delighted that he could help save his uncle's life. When Arthur pleaded with him to not sacrifice himself, Gawain said, "It is my choice and my decision. I will return with you tomorrow and agree to the marriage on condition that the answer she supplies is the correct one to save your life."

Arthur and Gawain met Lady Ragnell and agreed to her conditions. The next day, Arthur rode unarmed to meet Sir Gromer and at first, he gave him all the answers that he had collected from near and far. Sir Gromer held up his sword to cleave Arthur in two. Arthur added, "I have one more answer. What a woman desires above all else is the power of sovereignty—the right to exercise her own will." Sir Gromer, angered by the answer, knew that his stepsister had probably given him the correct answer and swore an oath against her as he ran off into the forest, sparing Arthur.

Gawain held to his promise and married Lady Ragnell when they arrived back at the castle that day. After the wedding feast, where all present were in shock at the horror of the monstrous bride that Gawain had married, the newlyweds retired to the wedding chamber. Lady Ragnell asked Gawain to kiss her. He went to her and kissed her and when he stepped back, saw the most beautiful young woman, smiling at him.

Gawain was taken aback and wary of her sorcery and asked what had happened to her to effect such a dramatic change. She told him that her stepbrother had always hated her and had told his mother who had knowledge of sorcery to cast a spell on her to change her into a monstrous creature. She could only be released by the spell if the greatest knight in Britain would willingly choose her for his bride. Gawain asked her why Sir Gromer hated her so much.

"He thought me bold and unwomanly because I defied him. I refused his commands both for my property and my person." Gawain smiled at her in admiration and marveled that the spell was now broken. "Only in part," she said. "You have a choice, my dear Gawain, which way I will be. Would you have me in this, my own shape at night and my former shape by day? Or would you have me grotesque at night in our chamber and my own shape in the castle by day? Think carefully before you choose."

Gawain thought for a moment and knelt before her, touched her hand and told her it was a choice that he could not make because it was her choice only to make. He told her that whatever she chose he would willingly support. Ragnell radiated with joy. "You have answered well, dearest Gawain, for your answer has broken Gromer's evil spell forever. The last condition he set has been met! For he said that if, after marriage to the greatest knight in Britain, my husband freely gave me the power of choice, the power to exercise my own free will, the wicked enchantment would be broken forever."

Lady Ragnell and Gawain were united in sacred marriage of two equals who had made a free and conscious choice to come together. Sir Gromer had bewitched her for asserting her will and protecting her sexuality, and Gawain gave her the freedom to transform her disfiguration. She had the ability to save the king, and Gawain had the wisdom to recognize the sovereignty of the feminine. Together they found healing love and wholeness.

This is a powerful account of the healthy feminine and masculine (Ragnell and Gawain) and the distorted or shadow feminine (Gromer's mother) and masculine (Gromer).

This story is enacted in our own lives every day as we live in a society that tells us that our sovereign voices are not acceptable.

"No" is not acceptable. In order to reclaim our power, we must have the courage to say it, to wander in "the forest" alone connected to our truth, and wait there without compromising ourselves. We must risk being labeled as "monstrous" or nonconformist due to our disobedience to the patriarchal "power principle." The healthy masculine will always seek union with the healthy feminine because wholeness is our natural state. We must first experience this intrinsically before it can manifest in our lives.

As nature continually moves towards balance and wholeness, our nature also moves us towards balance, awakening us to ways in which we can reintegrate the healthy masculine and feminine into our lives. For us, achieving wholeness requires consciousness and framework, and a trust in our process. When we view our life experiences through this lens, we will be able to experience the sacred more deeply.

9

Reframing Health Care

Faith dares the soul to go farther than it can see.
~William Clarke

Modern health care is an extension of our current cultural mythology. It stands on an unhealthy foundation and it operates from the wounded masculine through the "power principle." The Feminine Principle is nowhere in sight. The patient is the victim of the illness and the physician carries the expertise to fix it. The patient is dependent on the physician to fix the illness.

Healing is not accessible in the physician's office, where only expertise fixes. The patient arrives here expecting to be healed. The medical system purports to heal and frequently falls short of its promise. The marketing ads that use terms connected with healing are not engaged in the actual physician-patient relationship. The Feminine Principle is not a part of their fifteen minute office visit. In the exam room, the physician is rewarded for expertise, but not for healing. Healing takes time, presence and framework. Healing is a process.

Those who run the system and keep it financially lucrative are under the false assumption that *process* reduces financial gain. This assumption is driving the flawed framework of our *product*-oriented medical model. Patients feel disillusioned and disempowered in this system. They go their seeking answers to life's questions about their suffering and symptoms, and are dismissed with only prescriptions. Their conditioning would tell them that this is "normal" medical practice, but their hearts and feelings speak otherwise. Their unaddressed feeling function often drives them away from this system as it does not hold space for their process.

The medical system will need to balance its expertise with a healing presence (the Masculine with the Feminine Principle), if physicians are to be both therapeutically and cost effective. Cost effectiveness is a conflict of interest for the medical system that is sustained by the high cost of sick care. How can cost effective medicine be practiced in a system like this? This is a closed system. How can a closed system support a patient's process? These are dilemmas that our health care system needs to address. Patients expect physicians to help them answer some of life's most difficult questions. Patients are often ill and afraid, and sometimes at the end of their lives looking for comfort, solace, and a way to die peacefully. Prescriptions and procedures do not address these deep needs. Procedures are costly and palliate the medical system's fear of death which is perceived as a failure of expertise. The medical system needs a framework that engages the physician's presence and empowers patients to face illness and death. The physician's presence needs to hold space and bear witness to patients in order to reframe these definitions of life and death that the system has distorted.

The disempowered patient

Physicians also suffer from the absence of the sacred feminine in health care. Their inability to hold space for healing and to mirror it back to the patient has starved the soul of traditional medicine. They are not taught how to bear witness with heart or presence. Witnessing others in this way is a skill that takes time and mentoring to cultivate. The patient often leaves the physician's office with only prescriptions to cover symptoms originating in her deepest body. Her body does not stop delivering its deliberate message, and the time between doctor visits leaves her fearful of the unknown.

She becomes anxious and feels lost as a result of a medical framework that is not interested in the causes of her symptoms. She feels powerless and helpless with growing dependence on the physician's expertise that she expects to help her feel whole.

Alone in her process, she feels a lack of control over her life. Her biography is unimportant to the medical framework as this is not currently an area that traditional medicine values. The patient is without tools to find the causes of imbalance that have led to her symptoms and sometimes to her illness. She believes that illness is a random event that she cannot control, and unaware, she continues to live in ways that contribute to it. The system has deeply failed her. It has made her dependent on it, and as a result, she has become "a victim waiting to be rescued." This dynamic has been normalized by our society and has contributed to the cultural trance that keeps us asleep to the power that self-responsibility carries for our healing.

When women perceive themselves as victims of their illnesses, they abdicate their power and second-guess themselves. They perceive that the physician has the power to help them, as they are not experts and lack the understanding of why they are sick. With wounded instincts they are unable to trust in their inner knowing. They live within a culture where they are imprinted to think that there is no connection between their lifestyle and their health. In our quick-fix society, self-responsibility, empowerment and transformation are not valued. The traditional medical system does not teach physicians how to incorporate these values into their work. Women feel helpless because this system does not honor process. It does not acknowledge the labor and endurance needed for transformation. Women are left seek to answers to their questions on their own.

Imagine a medical system where its framework included an exploration of the Four Body System. Imagine it was committed to transformation, healing and process in addition to fixing symptoms. This system would be passionate about educating patients to understand how to live better and with harmony. It would seek the causes of illness in order to restore health. Imagine what it could feel like to live from consciousness, to make changes that facilitated health; where physicians were teachers, facilitators and coaches who empowered patients to explore ways of healing in addition to their expertise. We could have a very different health care system as well as a society of more conscious and self-responsible people.

In this system, *health* would be normalized rather than illness. With this framework, we could teach our children to dismantle the unhealthy conditioned behaviors that we modeled for them. By addressing deeper issues that lead to illness and disease, we could model a healthier way of living. We could trust in our process and live and die with consciousness. This could change the face of our suffering and provide solutions for our health care crisis.

The price of fear

Fear is bad for our health. Innumerable studies have shown how fear has negative effects on our immune system—it weakens it. A weak immune system is a set-up for illness. Our fear drives our unconscious patterns of behavior that affect health. It results in anxiety and depression and disconnects us from our intrinsic power. Fear drives our need for comfort foods that we use to self-medicate. Comfort foods harm our cell structure. Their soothing is temporary and they leave their footprint in our cells which stay stymied for a long time and weaken our biology. Comfort foods inflame our tissues and worsen anxiety.

When midlife women use food to medicate their menopausal symptoms, it worsens how they feel. This form of self-medication is toxic to the Four Body System and is also often accompanied by shame. When patients with cancer use food to self-medicate, they feed cancer cells leaving their bodies toxic and weak.

Fear is also a common feeling present in our medical system. Physician training does not include the patient's perspective patient and the value that empowerment carries in healing. In fact, fear is very much a part of the physician-patient interaction in medical training. Medical training imprints physicians to interact in ways that evoke fear in their patients. They are not conscious of this. Most live from their adapted selves during medical training and they learn what is mentored and taught by the closed system of medicine. For most patients, physicians carry the status of high priest or priestess, the exclusive expert, making predictions about life, death and health. This is common practice with cancer patients. Our culture has assigned the stigma of a "death sentence" to cancer. We have created this through our limited perception of its causes. We spend billions of dollars on cancer research, but there will never be a cure at the physical level of manifestation. A cure will require an understanding of *why* cancer manifests due to imbalances at *all* levels of the Four Body System, the toxic environment in which we live, and what is needed to restore balance and health. Waging war on the Physical body through pharmaceuticals or surgery does not cure it. All it does is palliate the cancer by temporarily removing it. Patients continue to be fearful of recurrence due to their lack of understanding of its causes.

It is difficult for patients to overcome a negative prognosis from the expert. When it is delivered, it permeates their unconscious and drains them of life energy. This does grave damage to their personal power and weakens their immune system. It activates hopelessness, depression, anxiety and causes intense fear. Patients put up "a good fight," but for most it is an "uphill battle," as they do not have an understanding of causes, or the knowledge needed in order to heal. Robert Johnson's statement, "The right treatment at the wrong level is ineffective," applies to the reason that patients are fearful. They fear the recurrence of their cancer due to the unaddressed levels from which the cancer originated. They live with the fear of premature death. Fear takes residence in their hearts and does not leave even after they are declared "cancer free" by the experts. Then they are merely "cancer survivors." The fear of recurrence always looms in the background. Fear sabotages their transformation into *true* health.

Those who do not accept the negative prognosis, often live long and healthy lives. They are known as "case reports," or "anecdotes" by the medical system. They are the ones worthy of study. They heal because they refuse the fear that is offered to them. They refuse to make cancer a part of their identity. Cancer can bring an acute awareness of the temporary nature of life. For people who view cancer from this perspective, their lives take on a deeper meaning and they live each day with this awareness. They begin to honor and value the power of self-responsibility and are able to make more conscious choices. Cancer can be a great teacher. It can paradoxically facilitate the pursuit of health and vitality within the people it affects. These courageous ones do not depend solely on the expertise of the closed system of traditional medicine. They use what it offers and enhance it with other disciplines in order to heal the multiple levels of imbalance. They seek, therefore they heal. They have learned how to prevent fear from influencing their outcomes. They are regenerative and resilient. They use both traditional methods and guidance from their inner wisdom resulting in better outcomes with traditional and complementary medicine. They balance both elements of the Masculine Feminine Principles.

They are the warriors of our society. They may have an "incurable" wound, but are able to deactivate its power by exploring its cause. Through self-responsibility, they reframe their lifestyles and their relationships to themselves, starving the causes of the cancer. They have reconfigured their health from an intrinsic place and their perspective does not allow for victimhood. They are not "cancer survivors." They have transcended survivorship and have *truly* healed.

Physicians need to be aware that the statistical prognoses that they share with patients lack accuracy. Statistical prognoses are averages. On either side of the statistical middle are extremes. On one extreme is success, and on the other is failure.

It would benefit all to focus on the side of positive outcomes and explore these methods in order to make recommendations for health and healing. Patients who heal are seekers. Physicians must explore ways that they can activate the seeker in order to increase positive outcomes in their patients. This is a sacred task for all. One ill patient cannot be compared to another. Everyone's health and illness is greatly influenced by their biology, biography, lifestyle, and the perspective. Physicians are trained in ways that disempower their patients and take away their hope. This is a critical issue that must be addressed. Physicians need to become aware of the fear they may be evoking in their patients and empower them instead. The elements of the Feminine Principle must be incorporated into both the medical system and the physician-patient encounter. The system must evolve into an open system free from fear. Empowerment must be weaved into office visits and prognoses must be delivered with a hope for healing. Physicians must learn strategies to help and heal their patients so their prognoses can improve as intrinsic power is accessed. In this way, both expertise and exploration will improve outcomes as well as patient health and compliance.

The medical system has a responsibility to educate patients about the levels of cause, to empower them to make healthier choices, and to encourage them to sustain these choices. It has a responsibility to engage patients in their healing process as a part of the solution to their illness. It also has a responsibility to heal the fear present in its patients because paralyzed immune systems cannot sustain health. Instead, the fear that is projected feeds unhealthy patterns that patients re-engage in order to feel better—the patterns that may have initially lead to their illness.

Our current health care system has become a part of the problem, not the solution. For patients and physicians to have any sense of meaning in their relationship to their health and work, these patterns must be uncovered and healed. The medical system must transform from the closed system it is currently, into an open one that can facilitate healing.

The inner life of the doctor

As health care became a closed system, physicians began to suffer. Physicians have been trained to help and heal. They cannot practice effectively within the closed system of medicine. They quickly discover that the system that employs them controls their medical decision making. They are intimidated into following protocols of productivity at the cost of their vocation. Process is not an option in their patient encounters, and the larger system of medicine regulates their performance. They are given fifteen minutes to fix their patients and they receive consequences from authorities if they take longer. They leave the exam room feeling saccharine accomplishment, and find superficial solace within organized medicine.

Physicians attempt to normalize this paradigm of the practice of medicine. But feelings don't lie, and month after month and year after year, the compromises that physicians feel within, deepen, holding them prisoners in the current superficial framework of profit driven, regulated health care. It regulates their methods and their ability to practice from soul. Health care itself has become superficial, adapted and empty. Physicians seek ways to comfort the emptiness they feel due to the lack of meaning in their work. They adapt to a system that is removed from the sacred vocation of *health*, *care*, and of healing itself, in order to survive.

The office visit revisited

The territory of the psyche changes in midlife. After half a lifetime, the emptiness and hunger from the emotionally starved self surfaces, and we begin to question the compromises we have normalized and mistaken for our real selves. We look for a safe space within which to validate our emotional hunger and our wounded feeling function. Many hope they can experience this in their physician's office as their symptoms that frighten them. Physicians need to be conscious their patient's needs in order to provide both comfort of their expertise and safety of their presence, to be able to hold a safe space for the patient's suffering and facilitate *true* healing. In order to provide this, physicians would need to be committed to their own personal growth, as they cannot offer their patients what they are not.

There is an old saying, "What happens to a person in your presence is more a matter of who you are than what you know." This truth is not taught in medical schools. Physicians are taught to become experts at the cost of their feeling function. This deprives their patients of true healing. In order for true healing to occur, physicians must be able to offer empathy and hold a safe space for the pain that their patients feel without invalidating it.

What the office visit can heal is the invalidated and wounded feeling function that patients bring to their encounter with the physician. For some, when a safe space is held, repressed feelings may emerge that can reconnect them with their real selves and bring balance to their Emotional bodies. For some this brings meaning back into their lives. As they heal their disconnection from their real selves, they can begin to trust the power and wisdom of their feeling function and can dismantle their adapted selves. A physician's ability to bear witness to patients with the power of their presence can often transform illness into health. Sometimes prescriptions are not even needed with this form of "medicine."

For the patient this is the sacred moment when she makes contact with answers to her crucial questions. She can uncover them in the partnership with her physician. She no longer feels alone in the world. This experience can also dismantle her fear. The patient can begin to trust in her process and look for creative solutions to reframe her life in order to restore her health. In this way, she can transform her experience of illness from one of chaos and disorder into one of order within the chaos that the illness has caused. Her illness calls her to reconfigure life from a real place within. Through this perspective, she can see how her choices contributed to the imbalances that led to her illness. She can use what she has learned and apply it to heal. She can begin to seek. This evokes self-responsibility. In this way, the patient's identification moves from the Victim to the Warrior. The Warrior mobilizes her life force in order to transform her and promote health.

How powerful would an office visit like this be for both the physician and the patient? This is a question worth asking and imagining. We fall short in our system without this question. Patient encounters are bereft of this level of meaning and physicians relate to patients' adapted selves from their adapted selves seeking what is familiar and conditioned. True safety can only be experienced in connection to the real self. This is what is missing in our medical system today. This is a framework worth reintegrating.

The Feminine and Masculine Principles revisited

It is worth restating that the elements of the Feminine Principle are creative and fecund. Fecundity is a characteristic of incubation. Incubation is necessary for creativity.

The elements of Masculine Principle analyze and fix. The Feminine when balanced with the Masculine Principle promotes wholeness. One without the other creates imbalance. Creative thought without action manifests nothing. Fixing without process does not heal. When we listen, validate, empower, educate and treat, there is greater opportunity for healing. The understanding of cause is critical for cure. A framework limited to the body remains incomplete.

Anxiety is often a result of the disempowered state. It results from fear; fear of death, loss, transformation and the unknown. The patient is not equipped with the tools needed to find order in the chaos that illness evokes. Physicians must offer these to her. These tools can uncover her ability to seek at all levels and learn about the inner transformation and healing that her illness can facilitate. Medicine practiced from this framework can reframe the patient's life and awaken her consciousness. She can then begin to question without fear. Her questions can help her make contact with what is real and meaningful for her. These questions can transform her life. This is a powerful medical framework that is sacred and pure. It is inclusive and open. It combines medical expertise with presence and process. The closed system of medicine does not support this. Physicians have not been trained to engage in this way in the exam room. Patients feel neglected and forgotten. They feel abandoned in their process.

A failing business model

Currently, we are a three trillion dollar health care system that has more debt than it has worth. The health care system is failing both as a vocation and a business. Both patients and physicians are disillusioned and adapting to the closed system of medicine. Country clubs, golf outings and pharmaceutical dinners add nothing of value to the physician's soul. Fear is boundless in patient rooms and physician offices. Physician burn-out coupled with increasing rates of alcohol and drug abuse are climbing every year. The feminine is buried and all of us are suffering from the symptoms of her absence.

As long we adapt to the current closed system of health care, it will continue its meaningless pursuit of profit over process. Those that do not adapt will continue to be ejected. A medical system controlled by those disconnected from its sacred vocation cannot possibly serve health. The soul of medicine cannot live when its mission is not being served. What is sacred to medicine is distant from corporate health care's quarterly profits.

Feeling function is critical in a healing paradigm

Emotion, energy in motion, engages imagination in the creative process. These elements of the Feminine Principle are not valued in our medical system. These elements need to be accessed in order for the current medical paradigm to transform into a more balanced and effective one.

> He who is badly wounded in his feeling function
> will not be happy over anything.
> ~Robert Johnson

It is the feeling function that gives meaning and worth to any system committed to the healing process. Without it, access to deep healing evades us. Our collective culture has a wounded instinct and feeling function. Patients and physicians are unhappy. Our system is in deep need of healing. Rearranging the furniture with health care reform only at the surface level of the current closed system of medicine will not heal it in the long run. It will not save money and will not serve the vocation of medicine until health care itself transforms into a more integrative and open system administered from a place that truly serves health, care and the healing process.

Integrative medicine revisited

The solution to our health care crisis may be through the implementation of a more inclusive and collaborative integrative medical model than the one that currently exists. It can no longer be a potpourri of traditional and complementary modalities that only physicians administer. It needs to engage the Four Body System in order to *truly* heal its patients. It cannot be used to lure market share. It must be engaged from the sacred intent of medicine. It must unite complementary with traditional medicine as an integrated whole, practiced with scientific method and standard of care, inclusive of the Feminine Principle. This is the only way that integrative medicine can truly heal patients and restore meaning to physicians.

There is great damage that the closed system of health care can do to integrative medicine. It may promote integrative medicine simply to attract market share, and when patients leave disillusioned, they may mistake their disappointing experience of it (within the current health care system) for the inefficacy of integrative medicine itself. The closed system of health care has distorted integrative medicine and expects it to follow the traditional rules of the closed system. Integrative medicine is unable to remain true to its purpose when practiced within the current closed system of health care.

Proscutes is a mythological character who cuts off the feet and head of his guests in order to accommodate the size of his bed. This is what is being done to integrative medicine within the current health care system. It has attempted to fit this open system into its closed system's box. It is also considered separate from the current model of health care. Integrative medicine is not meant to be a separate specialty within the current medical model. The current model needs to expand into an integrative model in order for it to be more effective. This inclusive model would combine both process and expertise without compromising standard of care. It would be cost effective and open to growth and healing. This has the potential to integrate both health and care back into health care.

True healing cannot be accessed without a framework that is inclusive of deeper levels of imbalance. This understanding is critical to reframing the current health care model. If we implement the current compromised framework of integrative medicine currently present in the medical system, we will create what we have now—a new specialty that is undervalued within traditional medicine, one that is an added cost to the patient.

In addition, physicians cannot offer standard of care medicine in complementary disciplines without in depth training. They need to practice the medicine in which they were originally trained. What they need is the training to address the *levels* that *cause* illness in order to triage patients to expert, complementary practitioners who can work at those levels. They can then work collaboratively with their expertise of the Physical body with practitioners who are experts in the Mental, Emotional and Energy bodies. Physicians need to use their tools responsibly in ways that maximize health and healing in their patients. We need to expand the medical system to be able to access the deeper levels of imbalance that can promote deeper levels of healing. In the long run, this will be less expensive and more effective than the current model of health care.

The Handless Maiden

I discovered the story of *The Handless Maiden*, after she appeared in a dream. As I began to explore its meaning, I became aware of the power of this story and its symbolic significance as it applied to our current health care system. It could be the story of the wounding that has occurred at the heart and soul of the vocation of medicine.

There was once a miller who had fallen on hard times. All he had left was a millstone and a large apple tree behind his mill. One day he was in the forest cutting deadwood and he came upon a charming man who said to him, "Why are you wasting your time cutting deadwood? I will make you wealthy beyond your wildest dreams and will come to claim what is behind your mill in three years." He then disappeared into the woods.

The miller thought nothing of it and wandered home. To his awe, he saw that his house was converted into a mansion with royal linens and draperies, the finest furniture and china. The miller's wife was overcome. "How did this happen?" she asked.

"I came upon a man in a black robe in the forest who promised me wealth and a life of ease in exchange for what is behind the mill. Surely we can plant another apple tree when he takes the one growing there now."

"Oh! Behind the mill is indeed an apple tree, but our daughter is there also, sweeping the yard. The man you met is the Devil."

The forlorn parents were devastated. The daughter did not marry for three years, and the day that the Devil came to collect her, she put on a white robe after she bathed and waited for him to take her.

When the Devil came to collect her, he began to scream, "She must not bathe or I cannot come near her." She then did not bathe for weeks and reeked of uncleanliness with matted hair and dirty clothes.

As the days passed, she began more and more to resemble a wild beast. But she wept hot tears that ran down her arms which cleared the dirt and left them white and clean.

When the Devil came to collect her, he was furious, "Chop off her hands, or I cannot come near her," he screamed. "If you don't, everything in your life will die."

The father was so frightened that he obeyed the Devil. He brought out his silver axe, and weeping and shaking, he begged forgiveness of his daughter and chopped off her hands. There was much crying out and the girl's life as she had known it had ended forever.

When the Devil returned to collect his bounty, the girl had cried so deeply that her stumps were clean and white as snow. The Devil was infuriated and could not take her away as her stumps were clean and he only wanted a dirty maiden.

The maiden then pleaded to her parents to let her leave and beg for food, and she went out wandering in the forest. It was a moonlit night and she wandered with her disheveled body and matted hair with the appearance of a wild beast with stumps wrapped in white gauze. She had left her parent's house and wandered into the woods to seek her destiny as the handless maiden. Pretty soon, she came upon a royal orchard where the pears on the trees shone silver in the moonlight. She knew that each was carefully counted, but she was so hungry that she begged the spirits of the tree for some fruit. A branch bent down for her and offered her a perfect pear. She ate it gratefully and returned to the forest to rest. The next day, the king came to his orchard and noticed a missing pear. He questioned the gardener who told him, "Last night, a girl without hands appeared and the tree offered her a pear as I watched."

The king brought his magician with him to watch if she would return that night. Indeed she returned at midnight and the tree again offered a branch to the handless maiden so she could eat the pear. The king was overcome by her beauty in the moonlight. He stepped out and declared himself to her and promised to care for her through all the days of her life. So the king married the handless maiden. He made her a set of silver hands to replace her absent hands.

A few years later, when the maiden was with child, the king had to go far away to wage a war and he left his mother in charge of her. He asked to be informed if the child was born in his absence. When the maiden gave birth, a messenger was sent to inform the king of the birth of the child. The messenger came to a river and stopped by the side of the water for a nap, as he felt tired. When he was asleep by the side of the river, the Devil switched the message, informing the king that the child was half beast. The king was horrified and sent a message back of love and caring for his wife and the deformed child. Again, the messenger fell asleep by the river and the Devil switched the message to read, "Kill the queen and her child." The Queen mother was devastated by this request and rather than follow the king's directive, strapped the baby on his mother's breast and bid her farewell, sending her into the forest.

The young queen wandered through the forest until she came upon a river. As she was parched and thirsty, she leaned forward to take a drink and her baby slipped out from its harness and fell into the river. The queen overcome by fright and love for her baby, suddenly thrust her stumps into the river and her hands instantly grew back. They grasped her baby and pulled him out of the river.

When the king got word that his queen had been sent out into the woods and that the messages had been changed through trickery, he went out into the deep woods to look for his queen and his child. He found them by the river and as they reunited, he rejoiced at their coming together again. They returned to the castle and lived a beautiful and fruitful life.

Despite all his efforts, the Devil was not able to destroy what was cleansed by tears and love.

This story is symbolic of the current state of health care in our country. The mill that processes raw material can be likened to our health care system. Since the mill is not working, symbolically health care has lost its ability to honor *process* and to include it as part of its framework. Of course, this is where the illness within the system begins. Rejection of process causes loss of vitality and abundance and the *real* work of medicine is not being done. The creative life within our current system is at a standstill and its true abundance has dried up. When we sacrifice our instincts, we find ourselves in situations where gold is promised, but grief is given in return. As a result, we are unable to see into the nature and the reality of things and we lose meaning in our work and in our lives.

Today, those who chose medicine as their vocation find themselves running on a treadmill with no way off, working for a heartless medical system. They cope through their adaptations in order to survive. Both patients and physicians experience a great loss of meaning. Patients come to the system for expertise and to experience the sacred feminine in their physician's presence. Physicians are not able to provide this for them. They are conditioned to discard elements of the Feminine Principle from the patient encounter. Due to its absence, patients are unable to connect with the healing gifts of their physicians and physicians are unable to heal their patients. When our instincts are cut off, our chances for error are heightened. Many physicians are not even aware of this. They have adapted to the absence of the Feminine Principle in their vocation as it is no longer considered a core value. Feeling function is dismissed as "touchy feely" or hysterical, and patients continue to leave their physician encounters with heart-break and fear. The "hands" of the system have been amputated.

Nearly twenty years ago, physicians made a Devil's bargain. The fathering function (protective aspect or vision-keeper) struck a Devil's bargain for financial gain and unknowingly betrayed the heart of their vocation. Physicians handed over the business of health care to the corporate world. When the fathering function, or vision-keeper, is unconscious of the soul compromises expected, a betrayal of the soul will occur. As a result, creativity and feeling will be cut off. As hands touch and sensate, they feel what conveys love and healing. A baby who is not touched fails to thrive. Illness cannot heal without the touch of the hands and heart. This has been proven in research studies on the power of healing touch. This function was abdicated by physicians by delegating the business of health care to business managers and accountants. In doing this, the vision of medicine was compromised and physician's sovereignty and their freedom to heal were abdicated in exchange for financial security. As physicians were not trained in business, they delegated it elsewhere. They lacked discernment. They did not realize the sorrow and anguish that this would cause. They did not think it would wound their calling to heal. This was a grave price to pay that hurt both physicians and patients. The system continues to grind on in the name of "health care," and projects the *illusion* of its mission through millions spent in advertising. It is promoting neither *health* nor *care*. Physician worth is determined by insurance companies who fail to reimburse for preventive medicine, and consequently fewer physicians are drawn into primary care. Primary care is no longer an affordable specialty for physicians. Subspecialties that are reimbursed more lucratively are becoming top heavy in the medical system. The promotion of true health has suffered greatly and we are all grieving its loss.

Our system is broken and no matter how shiny the silver hands are, they are not real. Without real hands, one is unable to function in feeling or instinct. We are all expected to suppress our pain of amputation and adapt to the closed system of medicine. This leaves all with great loss. No matter how much the masculine (the expert) is engaged, without the feminine (feeling), there can be no real health or healing.

Science, in its truest sense, is no longer practiced in medicine today. Increasingly, medicine has become a "crap shoot" where pharmaceuticals are dispensed without much thought in the hope that they will work. Prescribing is heavily influenced by pharmaceutical companies in their attempts to control physician practices for corporate profit.

The system, at this juncture, is "wandering in the woods with stumps wrapped in white gauze, holding its pure vocational seed against its chest, looking for comfort, for a drink of pure river water."

Current health care reform will not provide this. The Feminine Principle must be reintegrated with all of its elements. The skills of listening and feeling and the weaving of patients' stories with symptoms must all be allowed. The patient's pain and suffering must matter, and as patients and physicians hearts deepen with the presence of the sacred feminine, the vocation of medicine will heal.

The Devil must never be trusted. There is no real success without a joyful feeling function. If our rewards for productivity are numbers only, we will risk all that is of value to us. Physicians who are in midlife are no longer interested in silver hands. They want what is real and true to their hearts, where what they do matters and makes a difference to both themselves and their patients.

What the shock will be that forces them to thrust their "stumps" in the river out of love for their sacred work is anybody's guess, but it *will* happen, as the future can always be predicted from the path that the story takes.

The Devil will continue his efforts to tempt, and will be enraged by the feeling function when the sacred is restored into the vocation of medicine that is crying out for healing.

Health care is currently in crisis. To heal this, physicians need to reevaluate who they are, what they represent and for how long they will wander, holding close to their chests what they hold sacred and love deeply. For as long as physicians adapt to the conditions that the closed system creates for their work, they will be lost in the forest, far away from the healing river. Without soul, no system can be sustained, especially a system that purports to heal.

The illusion of health care is crumbling. Patients are going elsewhere for their healing. Physicians must awaken to this loss. They have put all that they value into their craft. Only physicians and patients can transform this. It will take great courage for them to individuate. Understanding and orientation are needed in order for them to know where they are in their process, so they can carefully and lovingly restore the heart of the vocation back to its true mission and vision. The medical system needs to dismantle its distortions and work authentically from its mission in order to be able to truly heal. It needs to reconnect and remember the creative and sacred feminine, so it can revive its soul.

We need physicians who are courageous, creative and able to recognize the emptiness they feel within when they are forced to adapt to what is not real in their work. Their compliance serves no one. They are no longer able to connect with their patients in ways that they dreamed, as laptop computers required to record patient encounters interfere with their presence in the exam room. The fear of error and imperfect documentation takes precedence over their ability to listen in order to effectively diagnose. What has become of the vision and vocation of medicine in the last two decades? Who would have thought this would happen? The accelerated pace with which the Feminine Principle is discarded from the system will push the soul of medicine deep underneath the weight of normalized layers of red tape. This will no doubt beckon an even deeper need for the system to deconstruct in order to heal its broken construct that requires the inclusion of the sacred feminine for achieving wholeness. Wholeness is the natural order of things. All of life moves towards wholeness. Illness is a stage in wholeness. Our medical system is currently ill. We must use the "medicine" we know to heal its broken heart as it makes its way towards becoming whole.

In medicine today, when physicians are called upon to add elements of the feminine, they often react from a place of *learned helplessness.* They mock and dismiss them as unimportant accessories that they believe interfere with their expertise. What they need to remember is that these elements can do much to heal the current imbalances within the system that is clearly taking health care off course. Consciousness is necessary and vital for a course correction in medicine and it will take courage and love to heal this sacred vision. Physicians need to reframe their current system and include elements of the Feminine Principle in order to restore meaning to their work. This is not exclusive of expertise. The health care system needs to individuate. This individuation will require the restoration of the sacred by its physicians and patients that comprise its heart and its soul.

The healing process never stops. The healer and the healed participate in a sacred partnership that must return to its original roots, its vocational intent. Without this, the shock of remembering health care's true mission will come as a crisis of collapse, where a system based solely on fear and profit will implode due to its disconnection from what is real.

Women's Health and the current medical model

When the Feminine Principle is absent in health care, women accessing it are not honored or served. Their cries and longings are not heeded. They are silenced with medications as the feminine skills of listening, learning, loving, transforming and process are ignored.

Women are left as they are today, with shame towards their feeling function, repressed and regressed, without guidance through their sacred initiation in midlife.

A woman at this medial juncture is transitioning from mother to crone. Her initiation into her role as a leader, teacher, mentor and a wise one is threatened by the system's inability to hold a safe and healing space for her. The system has a sacred task to help her reintegrate meaning and health into the second half of her life. If it does not perform this, she will live her remaining days with emptiness, and feel betrayed by her changing body, wishing for nature to turn back her clock. She will be unable to grow old gracefully with wisdom, joy, consciousness and health.

This is what is at stake. Our culture has distorted and betrayed what is real. I believe that we, as a collective, are sicker because of our disconnection from soul. We have struck a Devil's bargain, replacing what is real, soulful and creative with silver hands. We think that material success and corporate profit can fill the void left by our soul loss. This is simply not working.

Our elderly are discarded; our adults are disoriented; our children are living out of our shadows and our economy is failing. There is violence, suffering and lack of meaning wherever we turn.

We are the ones who can change this. It is up to us to find solutions that are intrinsic, in order to redefine and reframe what we have lost. Restoring the simple elements that bring us joy, fulfillment, love and connection is deeply needed. This is not rocket science. Waiting for a messiah, a president or an organization to change this will continue to place us in the role of the "victim waiting to be rescued." This is *our* task and we need to grow up and wake up to the story in which we are currently living and to give it a happy ending. It is up to *us* to rewrite our story, to understand the price of self-betrayal, the price of delegating our power and sovereignty to a value system bereft of heart and soul and feeling.

It is up to us to live more authentically and to use our voices to reclaim our birthright for wholeness, for health and for what is real and true. It is only then that we can truly heal. This is a process in which we all must participate. Our silence will continue to perpetuate our conditioned cultural patterns of learned helplessness.

Healing the health care system

As midlife women, we need to empower ourselves with the voice of our "double." It is strong and true and has a tone that is fierce and deep. It is connected to the truth of all things. As we connect to it and become who we really are, we will gain the insight and strategy to look for healing through our understanding of the causes for our illness.

Today, women are the main consumers of health care. The midlife woman, who is connected with what is real, is able to demand what is her right and privilege from the health care system. If her needs are not met, she will leave and look elsewhere for what she seeks. Her needs are simple and the framework she craves is one that can orient her in her life's gateway to a richer and larger relationship with herself. If we, in midlife, do not answer this call, we will have betrayed our sacred responsibility to transform our world for our future. We must all do our part. We must support and love each other into doing this.

Health care needs to be examined from the inside out, from the top down and the bottom up. There must not be any stone left unturned. When physicians analyze the current system in ways in which they were trained to analyze the body, they will be able to identify the pathology that keeps it sick. They will have to reach deep inside and stand in the face of criticism and rejection, with courage and heart so they can reconfigure the infrastructure of their sacred system that has lost its soul.

For the patient, this will mean looking for a physician who can meet her needs at all levels, who can honor her and her process with both expertise and presence. It will mean having the courage to speak her truth, and to expect a level of communication that fulfills her needs and provides her with education, healing, and standard of care medicine.

For physicians, it may mean practicing medicine from both heart and meaning. If the system cannot support this, it may mean practicing alone, until their patients support their uncompromising commitment to the vocation of medicine. It will mean creating an *open* system, where physicians incorporate an expanded view of health and illness by learning ways to offer their patient's strategies for healing that transcend traditional medicine.

In the midst of this crisis, lobbyists and politicians want to wish our problems away. They too, look for superficial solutions for symptomatic relief. They often create the *illusion* of change by offering quick-fixes and cover-ups that are short-lived and skin-deep. Their energy is mostly engaged in bipartisan struggles where the need for transformation is compromised in favor of personal gain and party support. The soul of the system can only be healed by its physicians and its patients and by no one else.

The health care system itself, top heavy with many layers of management and red tape, overcharges its patients and over-controls its physicians. It televises advertisements that create the *illusion* of health and wellness, of healing and well-being and of integrative medicine, thinking that the public will naively believe its efforts are sincere. But our public today consists of an overwhelming number of midlife women who will not be fooled into supporting a system that is not delivering what is real.

As we commit our lives to what is real, our world will no doubt be transformed for the better. In my least optimistic moments, when I worry about what my children will inherit, I gain solace in knowing that in our world, close to one billion midlife women are in process. They are hungry for a better world. They are hungry for what is real. Their appetites will not be satisfied by anything less than what resonates with truth and integrity. These are the ones who will change the face of health care and all the other organizations that are limping along without the Feminine Principle.

These are the ones we can count on to transmute the mess of our world into one of depth and wisdom and into one of value and love. We each have a powerful feeling function that speaks the language of our truth. We feel when we are being fooled, and we feel when we are being served. We will feel our way into behaving in ways that create a better world for our future. We are now called to become our "double" and She is awakening within our voices and our hearts. We have come to the end of the time when we are expected to adapt out of fear. The time has come for us to stand in the heat of transformation until our collective process is complete.

The solutions to our problems are not complicated. They are simple. We are called to open our hearts and our minds, and with that our systems, into a new paradigm of health care and Women's Health, one that functions from truth and meaning, love and creativity, expertise, and presence. Health care herself needs to heed the call of her "double." She is the one who has been waiting to restore her soul, the one who is restless and will not rest until Her system is transformed into one of truth and authenticity—the one whose healing beckons and the one whose time has come.

I invite you all to entertain these questions, to question the reality you are presented in your experience of today's health care system and to trust in your feeling function. Your "double" is always present, waiting for your connection, waiting to be lived in the new, authentic you. She has wisdom and instinct and She is always right. She is the voice of transformation and truth and will connect you to what is real. I invite you all to live out of Her and in doing so together we will transform our world.

Resources

The Ommani Center for Integrative Medicine,
   www.ommanicenter.com

Venessa Rahlston, Soul Genesis,
   www.soulgenesis.com

Healing Arts by Margaret,
   www.healingartsite.com

Diane Herold, Reiki Master and Teacher, Flower Essence Therapist,
   414-481-8569.

For a list of Compounding Pharmacies, please visit
   www.ommanicenter.com

Institute of HeartMath,
   www.heartmath.org

Dunn+Associates Design,
   www.dunn-design.com

Dorie McClelland,
   www.springbookdesign.com

Bibliography

Alkhalaf, M. et al. *Growth Inhibition of MCF-7 human breast cancer cells by progesterone is associated with cell differentiation and phosphorelation of Akt protein.* European Journal of Cancer Prevention, 2002 Oct; 11(5):481–8.

Beinfield, Harriet and Korngold, Efrem. *Between Heaven and Earth.* New York: Ballantine Books, 1991.

Campbell, Joseph. *The Hero with a Thousand Faces.* New Jersey: Princeton University Press, 1973.

Childre, Doc and Deborah Rozman. *Transforming Stress: The Heartmath Solution for Relieving Worry, Fatigue and Tension.* California: New Harbinger Publications. 2005.

Colditz, Graham A, et.al. *The Use of Estrogens and Progestins and the Risk of Breast Cancer in Postmenopausal Women.* The New England Journal of Medicine. 1995. Vol. 332(24): 1589–93.

Estes, Clarissa Pinkole. *Mother Night. Myths, Stories, and Teachings for Learning to See in the Dark.* Sounds True, Inc., 2010.

Estes, Clarissa Pinkole. *Women Who Run With the Wolves.* New York, Ballantine Books: 1992.

Hersmeyer, K., et al. *Reactivity-based coronary vasospasm independent of atherosclerosis in rhesus monkeys.* Journal of the American College of Cardiology. 1997. 29 (March 1): 671.

Holford, Patrick. *The New Optimum Nutrition Bible.* Berkeley, CA: The Crossings Press, 2004.

Johnson, Robert A. *We, Understanding the Psychology of Romantic Love.* San Francisco: HarperCollins Publishers, 1983.

Johnson, Robert, A. *Transformation, Understanding the Three Levels of Masculine Consciousness.* San Francisco: HarperCollins Publishers, 1991.

Judith, Anodea. *Eastern Body Western Mind.* Berkeley, CA: Celestial Arts Publishing, 1996.

Jung, Carl G. *Collected Works of C.G. Jung. Translated by R.F.C. Hull.* Princeton: Princeton University Press, 1972.

Lee, John and Hopkins, Virginia. *Dr. John Lee's Hormone Balance Made Simple.* New York: Wellness Central Hachette Book Group, 2006.

Lee, John and Hopkins, V. *What Your Doctor May Not Tell You About Menopause.* New York: Wellness Central Hachette Book Group, 2004.

Murdock, Maureen. *The Heroine's Journey.* Boston, MA: Shambala Publications, 1990.

Satir, Virginia. *Peoplemaking.* CA: Science and Behavior Books Inc., 1972.

Stein, Murray (editor). *Jungian Psychoanalysis.* Illinois: Opencourt Books, 2010.

Tool. Vicarious. *10,000 days.* Volcano Records. 2006.

Women's Health Initiative Study. *Risks and Benefits of Estrogen Plus Progestin in Healthy Postmenopausal Women.* JAMA, July 17, 2002.

Xiao, Ou Shu et.al. *Soy Food Intake and Breast Cancer Survival.* JAMA 2009: 302(22): 2437–2443.

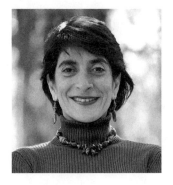

Kalpana (Rose) M. Kumar, M.D. is board-certified in internal medicine. She graduated from The Albert Einstein College of Medicine and completed her internship and residency in internal medicine at The University of California San Francisco and Stanford University Medical Center.

Her groundbreaking integrative medical framework has facilitated true healing for thousands of patients over the past 20 years. She is the founder and medical director of The Ommani Center for Integrative Medicine in Pewaukee, Wisconsin.

Dr. Kumar is an expert in the fields of Integrative Medicine, Women's Health and Executive Stress Reduction. She is a national speaker and health care consultant. She is a futurist and visionary who can offer innovative solutions to our current health care crisis.